CONTENTS

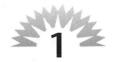

HEALING FOODS, HERBS AND VITAMINS

FOODS THAT CAN IMPROVE YOUR HEALTH

Source: The late **Maureen Salaman,** international nutrition and health lecturer. She authored *Foods That Heal.* Bay to Bay Distribution.

A growing body of scientific research shows that many natural foods contain vital nutrients that can help you stay well or regain your health. The greatest benefit is usually obtained when these foods are eaten in a close-to-natural state—raw or only lightly cooked—because our digestive tracts are designed to absorb nutrients from uncooked food.

Always be cautious about eating manmade, imitation foods because processing removes vital nutrients and adds many substances that can trigger food sensitivities and allergies.

Here are just a few of the diseases and unhealthy conditions that can be treated effectively or, better still, prevented, by good nutrition…

• *Arthritis.* Traditional medicine can give little help—other than painkilling drugs—to the estimated 23 million Americans who suffer from rheumatoid arthritis and osteoarthritis.

More than 1,000 years ago American Indians learned that the juice of the yucca plant could relieve arthritic pain. Modern research shows that *saponin* (the scientific name for yucca juice) protects friendly intestinal bacteria that compete with harmful microorganisms and prevent them from causing allergic reactions associated with arthritis. Yucca is available from health food stores.

OTHER WAYS ARTHRITIS IS RELIEVED: Reduced consumption of fat, increased intake of folic acid, protein, zinc, vitamins C and D, pantothenic acid.

• *Bad breath.* It usually originates in the stomach or intestinal tract, where food is incompletely digested because of a deficiency in hydrochloric acid.

SIMPLE SOLUTION: Take a tablespoon of apple cider vinegar before meals.

• *Bruising.* This can indicate a deficiency in vitamins C or K, bioflavonoids or zinc.

• *Cataracts.* They can develop when proteins in the eye lens are exposed to many years of oxidation and light. The process can be hastened by deficiencies in vitamins C, B-2 and D and the mineral calcium.

• *High cholesterol.* Drugs used to reduce cholesterol in the blood have a variety of dangerous side effects, but natural ways can be both safe and pleasant. **EATING THE SUGGESTED AMOUNTS OF THE FOLLOWING FOODS CAN HELP REDUCE CHOLESTEROL SIGNIFICANTLY...**

• Two or three apples a day.

• A serving of barley in hot or cold cereal or in baked goods several times a week.

• One cup of navy or pinto beans a day.

• Three medium carrots daily.

• Half or a whole green plantain daily.

• Three cups of yogurt a day.

• *Colds.* They can occur less often, be less severe and shorter-lived if you take vitamin C. *Other cold fighters:* Vitamins A, B-complex and E and zinc. Don't forget chicken soup.

CAUTION: More than 200 IU of vitamin E may be dangerous. Ask your doctor for the dose that's right for you.

• *Depression.* Mental depression is not only a result of emotional problems, it is often related to nutritional deficiencies.

AT RISK: Women depleted of essential nutrients by menstruation, childbirth or the use of birth control pills.

HELPFUL: Folic acid, vitamins B-6 and B-12, zinc and proteins.

Other nutrition-related contributors to depression are a vitamin C deficiency and food allergies.

• *Fatigue.* Many of us feel too tired most of the time to do very much. There are a variety of nutritional causes for this condition...and healthy eating can give us back our *joie de vivre.*

• *Epstein-Barr Syndrome and mononucleosis.* These two conditions are associated with overwhelming chronic exhaustion. They can be combatted with massive doses of vitamin C, followed by exercise.

OTHER HELPFUL NUTRIENTS: Vitamin A, chromium, manganese, selenium, zinc.

• *Gout.* Excruciatingly painful inflammation in the big toe and other joints—caused by crystallized uric acid—can be relieved, usually within a week or two, by eating six to eight cherries a day.

ANOTHER THERAPY: Three or more quarts of water daily.

• *Hypertension.* High blood pressure is called the "silent killer" because there are no external symptoms of the internal damage it wreaks on blood vessels. It leaves victims susceptible to stroke, heart failure and kidney damage. *The many causes of hypertension can include the following nutritional factors:* Excessive sodium, deficiency of potassium, calcium or magnesium, soft drinking water, refined sugar.

• *Osteoporosis.* Bones that have become weak and honeycombed often accompany aging. But this is not inevitable.

HELPFUL: More calcium, together with a moderate intake of vitamin D.

CAUTION: A high intake of protein (more than 100 grams a day) and too much phosphorus can cause calcium loss.

• *Prostate enlargement.* Common in older men, prostate enlargement can be reversed by increasing dietary zinc. You can get a sufficient amount from two ounces of herring, a lamb chop, two ounces of wheat germ, sesame seeds or soybeans, three ounces of chicken or a bowl of oatmeal.

• *Tooth and gum problems.* Conventional dental wisdom holds that tooth decay starts with diseased gums. However, recent research tells a different story. A bodily deficiency in calcium will draw calcium out of the jaw, causing loose teeth and inflamed gums.

SOLUTION: Increase your calcium intake. New bone formation can also be encouraged by taking vitamins A, C and D, magnesium and zinc.

HINT: If you grind your teeth when you sleep, you may stop naturally if you increase your calcium and pantothenic acid intake.

Best sources of nutrients...

• *Chromium.* Thyme (highest), black pepper, whole wheat.

• *Folic acid.* Torula (highest) and brewer's yeast, alfalfa, endive, chickpeas, oats.

• *Iodine.* Kelp (highest), cod liver oil.

• *Iron.* Kelp (highest), kidney, caviar, pumpkin and sesame seeds, wheat germ, blackstrap molasses, liver.

• *Manganese.* Tea leaves, cloves, ginger, buckwheat, oats, hazelnuts, chestnuts.

• *Pantothenic acid.* Royal jelly (highest), brewer's and torula yeast, brown rice.

• *Potassium.* Bananas, broccoli, avocado, Brussels sprouts, cauliflower, potatoes (with skins), cantaloupes, dates, prunes.

• *Protein.* Meat, poultry, fish, eggs, milk, nuts, beans, peas.

• *Selenium.* Corn, cabbage, whole wheat, beans.

• *Vitamin A.* Cod liver oil (highest), sheep and beef liver (they each have twice as much as calf's liver), carrots, yams.

• *Vitamin B-2.* Torula (highest) and brewer's yeast, liver, alfalfa, almonds.

• *Vitamin B-6.* Brewer's yeast, brown rice, whole wheat, soybeans, rye, lentils.

• *Vitamin B-12.* Liver (highest), sardines, mackerel.

• *Vitamin D.* Sardines, salmon, tuna, egg yolk, sunflower seeds.

• *Vitamin E.* Wheat germ (highest by far), safflower nuts, sunflower seeds, whole wheat.

• *Zinc.* Herring (highest by far), sesame seeds.

■

THE ANTIOXIDANT REVOLUTION

Source: **Kenneth H. Cooper, MD, MPH,** president and founder of the Cooper Aerobics Center, Dallas, which includes the Cooper Clinic and the Institute for Aerobics Research. He is author of *Dr. Kenneth H. Cooper's Antioxidant Revolution.* Thomas Nelson Publishers.

Antioxidants are invisible allies in our drive to improve health. They are good scavenging molecules that ride the bloodstream, gobbling up molecules of unstable oxygen called *free radicals.* The oxygen is called free because each molecule is seeking another molecule to cling to.

Free radicals are good in that they kill bacteria, help fight inflammation and control the tone of the smooth muscles, which regulate the blood vessels and internal organs. The problem starts when hordes of them run wild. **UNCHECKED FREE RADICALS...**

- *Injure the lenses of the eyes,* causing cataracts.

- *Harm skin tissue,* fostering premature signs of aging.

- *Change, through oxidation, the particles of low-density lipo-protein (LDL) into bad cholesterol* in the walls of blood vessels so that white blood cells can't destroy them. The result is a gradual buildup of plaque inside the artery walls that can lead to heart disease, strokes and heart attacks.

- *Enter individual cells, damaging the nucleus and the genetic code (DNA) it contains.* The damaged cell can become part of a cancerous lesion or tumor.

Internal antioxidants cling to free radicals, stopping their forays into tissue. But aspects of modern life tend to create too many free radicals for endogenous antioxidants to defuse. You can counter that overload by reducing your exposure to free radicals and adding more external (exogenous) antioxidants to your defenses. **AMPLIFY YOUR ANTIOXIDANT POWER WITH THREE SIMPLE STEPS...**

- *Consume the right amounts of certain vitamins* through a combination of food and daily supplements.

- *Engage in frequent moderate exercise.*

- *Make your home, work and recreational environments as healthy as possible.*

DAILY ANTIOXIDANT DIET...

My dietary recommendations start with the standard ones.
- *Eat as little fat as possible,* especially animal fat.
- *Include plenty of grains and fresh fruits.*
- *Avoid fried foods.*
- *Steam, don't boil, vegetables, and eat lots of them,* especially broccoli, Brussels sprouts, cabbage, cauliflower, spinach and collard greens.
- *In addition, take a daily "antioxidant cocktail"* (in pill form) of vitamin C, vitamin E and beta-carotene (a precursor—provitamin—of vitamin A).* Vitamin A itself can be toxic in large amounts. And the foods that contain it—liver, butter, eggs— are loaded with fat and cholesterol.

Health professionals often claim that you can get all the nutrients you need from a balanced diet. For some nutrients, that's true, although it would require you to eat, say, 15 oranges a day to consume enough vitamin C...or three cups of butternut squash for beta-carotene.

A sufficient quantity of vitamin E would be loaded with fat and calories—a cup of sunflower seeds or almost seven cups of peanuts.

For about $6 a month, the "cocktail" will...
- *Protect you against many forms of cancer.*
- *Build stronger defenses against cardiovascular disease* (hardened arteries, heart attack, stroke).
- *Help prevent cataracts and macular degeneration* (a major cause of blindness for people older than 65 years of age).
- *Delay the onset of premature aging.*
- *Boost your immune system.*
- *Reduce your risk of developing early Parkinson's disease.*

All this is true even if your cholesterol profile doesn't improve.

I recommend that daily supplements total...
- *Vitamin E:* 400 IU (international units—approximately equal to 400 milligrams [mg]).*
- *Vitamin C:* 1,000 mg twice a day, split into two doses.
- *Beta-carotene:* 25,000 IU (approximately equal to 15 mg).

To pursue athletic fitness, regularly achieving more than 80% of your predicted maximum heart rate during exercise

*Due to the possible interactions between vitamin E and various drugs and supplements, as well as other safety considerations, be sure to consult your doctor before starting a vitamin E regimen.

...or if you weigh more than 200 pounds, daily supplements could total...
- *Vitamin E:* 1,200 IU.
- *Vitamin C:* 2,000 mg (women), 3,000 mg (men), split into two or three doses.
- *Beta-carotene:* 50,000 IU.

Taking the full amount indicated here beyond what's contained in your food is safe for most people, but check with your doctor to be sure.

POSSIBLE SIDE EFFECTS...

If you take blood thinners (anticoagulants such as aspirin or Coumadin) for heart problems, have your blood tested once or twice a year for cholesterol and other lipids (fatty elements in the blood). Supplemental vitamin E could raise your lipid levels.

Vitamin C tablets can dissolve tooth enamel if chewed. Swallow them. And don't take more than 4,000 mg a day...too much can cause diarrhea and increase the risk of kidney stones.

Beta-carotene supplements may be unwise for people who smoke more than a pack of cigarettes a day. They may also cause liver damage if combined with an ounce or more of pure alcohol daily (two four-ounce glasses of wine or one mixed drink).

Anyone who has recently had surgery...who is extremely overweight...or who has a chronic condition such as diabetes or heart disease must obtain a doctor's approval before making a radical change in diet or exercise.

FREEDOM FROM FREE RADICALS...

While fighting free radicals created by oxidating foods, your body must also combat free radicals caused by the environment. These free radicals seem to encourage the inflammation of muscles, ligaments and joints that have already sustained injuries from sports or accidents, arthritis and other long-term conditions.

Take steps to minimize or eliminate your exposure to...
- *Your own and others' cigarette smoke.* It promotes lung cancer and early signs of aging, such as wrinkled skin.
- *Air pollutants* like smog, ozone, vehicle exhaust and chemicals in factories. These have direct links to diseases of the heart and lungs, including lung cancer.

• *Ultraviolet rays* from sunlight or sunlamps that emit those rays (not all do).

• *Total radiation* from electromagnetic fields, emitted by high-voltage wires...televisions...electric blankets...computers...microwave ovens.

SHORT-TERM STRATEGY: Don't try to change your life all at once. Start with your biggest problem. If you smoke, or someone in your home smokes, that's the best place to start.

LONG-TERM STRATEGY: Describe in writing the environments associated with all your regular activities for one week. Deliberately reduce your exposure to free radicals in each case.

∎

GREEN TEA: THE ULTIMATE ANTIOXIDANT

Source: **Lester A. Mitscher, PhD,** distinguished professor of medicinal chemistry at the University of Kansas in Lawrence. He is coauthor of *The Green Tea Book.* Penguin.

Antioxidants are remarkable compounds that fight disease by blocking cellular damage caused by highly reactive molecular fragments called *free radicals*.

Produced in the body by exercising, breathing polluted air and/or taking certain drugs, free radicals have been blamed for heart disease, cancer and other serious ailments.

STRONGEST ANTIOXIDANT...

Researchers have identified many different antioxidants, including vitamins A, C and E and the mineral selenium. Until recently, however, no one knew *which* antioxidant had the most potent disease-fighting effect.

Now one clear winner has emerged. It's *epigallocatechin gallate* (EGCG), a compound that belongs to a family of antioxidants known as *polyphenols*.

EGCG and other polyphenols are constituents of tea—especially of *green* tea. **THIS REMARKABLE BEVERAGE...**

• *Lowers levels of LDL (bad) cholesterol and keeps LDL cholesterol from undergoing oxidation.* The fatty deposits (plaques) that form along the artery walls of heart disease sufferers are caused by oxidized LDL cholesterol.

One study found that total cholesterol levels of men who drank five cups of green tea a day were nine points lower than those of men who didn't drink green tea.

• *Lowers blood pressure and inhibits blood clotting.* These benefits have a significant impact on cardiovascular health.

Studies have shown that several cups of green tea a day can cut an individual's risk for heart disease and stroke in half—even among people who have already experienced one stroke.

• *Interferes with cancer cells.* By rendering cellular DNA resistant to mutation, green tea prevents cancer cells from forming and inhibits the growth of tumors already in existence.

Green tea shows special promise against cancers of the stomach, esophagus, bladder, colon, pancreas and lung. Used in ointment form, it even seems to block the development and progression of skin cancer.

• *Enhances immunity.* Green tea boosts the activity of a number of key immune system components, including B-cells, T-cells and natural killer cells.

Green tea is especially beneficial for people undergoing chemotherapy, since chemo agents tend to lower counts of immune system cells.

• *Facilitates digestion.* It does so by encouraging the growth of beneficial bacteria in the intestine...and by controlling levels of glucose in the bloodstream.

• *Prevents tooth decay.* As long as it's held in the mouth for a few seconds before being swallowed, green tea helps reduce levels of dental plaque.

BOTTOM LINE: People who drink green tea on a daily basis have unusually low rates of heart disease and cancer. They also live longer. And unlike other antioxidants, those in green tea cause no toxic side effects.

GREEN TEA VS. BLACK TEA...

Both green and ordinary black tea are made from the same plant *(Camellia sinensis).* But green tea is *far* more healthful.

REASON: Because green tea undergoes less processing than black tea, it contains twice the concentration of polyphenols. One cup of green tea contains 300 to 400 milligrams (mg), compared with about 150 to 200 mg per cup of black tea.

Green tea contains roughly one-third less caffeine than black tea.

GREEN TEA DOSAGES...

Even one cup a day is beneficial. For maximum benefit, however, studies suggest that it's better to drink four cups a day.

This recommendation is backed up by population studies conducted in Asia, where the average person consumes four to six cups of green tea per day...and where rates of heart disease and cancer are remarkably low.

IMPORTANT: Antioxidant activity peaks about 30 minutes after drinking the tea. To keep levels of EGCG at consistently high levels, space the cups several hours apart.

If you don't like the taste of green tea, consider green tea capsules, sold in drugstores. One capsule is roughly equivalent to four cups of green tea.

DRAWBACK TO CAPSULES: They provide a large "pulse" of antioxidants rather than a sustained dose. And unlike tea, the capsules do *not* help prevent dental problems.

BUYING GREEN TEA...

Green tea is sold in health food stores and in supermarkets. Some brands are imported from China, others from Japan. Both varieties contain high levels of polyphenols.

Be sure to get the highest grade tea available. High-grade tea contains higher concentrations of antioxidants than low-grade tea. (The grade of a tea refers to the degree of leaf fragmentation—the less broken the leaf, the higher its grade.)

ALSO IMPORTANT: Freshness. The longer green tea sits on a shelf, the lower its antioxidant potency. Fresh green tea leaves are light yellow or light green. A brownish hue means the tea has undergone oxidation, which destroys antioxidants.

TO PREVENT OXIDATION: Store tea in an airtight container. If you buy tea bags instead of loose tea, make sure they are individually wrapped in foil.

BREWING GREEN TEA...

Drop one teaspoon of loose tea or a tea bag into a cup of freshly boiled water. Cover the cup with a lid, and let it steep for five minutes before drinking.

CAUTION: A shorter steeping time means you won't get the maximum dose of antioxidants. If the tea steeps for more than five minutes, the antioxidant compounds will start to degrade. Don't reuse tea bags or leaves.

■

VITAMIN THERAPY REDUCES SENILITY RISK

Source: **Hannes Stahelin, MD,** chairman, department of geriatrics, University Hospital, Basel, Switzerland. His 20-year study of 442 men and women, 65 to 95 years of age, was published in the *Journal of the American Geriatrics Society,* 12012 S. Compton Ave., Suite 313, Los Angeles 90059.

The risk of senility can be reduced via long-term vitamin therapy. Men and women who had a high intake of food rich in vitamin C or beta-carotene or who had taken supplements of vitamin C and beta-carotene for at least 20 years scored higher on memory function tests than did similar adults who had low vitamin levels. *Theory:* These antioxidant vitamins protect brain cells from damage by free radicals.

■

HERBAL HELP FOR PMS

Source: The late **Varro E. Tyler, PhD,** professor emeritus of pharmacognosy at Purdue University, West Lafayette, IN. He authored *Tyler's Herbs of Choice: The Therapeutic Use of Phytomedicinals.* Haworth Press.

Folklore has it that monks used the peppery fruit of the chasteberry bush *(Vitex agnus-castus)* to suppress their sexual desires.

Today chasteberry is used by women as a natural remedy for premenstrual syndrome (PMS) and other ailments caused by hormone imbalances.

Support for the use of chasteberry comes from a distinguished panel of German scientists, who recently completed a lengthy review of research on herbal remedies.

The panel recommended chasteberry for bloating, headache, depression and other symptoms of PMS...for menopausal hot flashes...and for painful breasts.

Chasteberry acts on the pituitary gland, a pea-sized gland located at the base of the brain. In turn, the pituitary gland signals the ovaries to restore a normal balance of the hormones estrogen and progesterone.

If you'd like to try chasteberry, consult your doctor to be sure that your symptoms stem from a hormone imbalance.

For PMS, chasteberry generally should be taken from the onset of symptoms until the beginning of the menstrual period.

For other problems, chasteberry can be taken continuously for up to six months.

The usual dose is 20 milligrams (mg) per day. To avoid side effects—typically, mild gastrointestinal problems such as nausea —take chasteberry with meals.

CAUTION: Chasteberry should be avoided by women who are pregnant or on hormone therapy.

Chasteberry is available in health food stores as a liquid extract or in capsule form.

■

MAXIMUM IMMUNITY: PROVEN METHODS FOR BOOSTING YOUR BODY'S DISEASE-FIGHTING POWER

Source: **Leo Galland, MD,** director, Foundation for Integrated Medicine, New York City. His latest book is *The Fat Resistance Diet.* Broadway. *www.fatresistance diet.com.* Dr. Galland is a recipient of the Linus Pauling award.

From cancer to the common cold, illness and infection are kept at bay by your immune system. **HERE'S HOW TO MAKE YOUR IMMUNE SYSTEM AS STRONG AS IT CAN BE...**

IMMUNITY-BOOSTING FOODS...

The average American gets about 30% of daily calories from cookies, potato chips and other snacks.

These and other nutrient-poor foods—including fast food—displace the nutrient-dense foods that the immune system needs to stay healthy.

FOR OPTIMAL IMMUNITY: Have two servings of fruit and five or six servings of vegetables each day.

In addition to vitamins and minerals, fruits and vegetables contain hundreds of *phytochemicals.* These natural substances protect cells against the damaging effects of free radicals...and boost the synthesis of carcinogen-neutralizing enzymes.

Phytochemicals include...

• *Allyl sulfides.* Found in onions and garlic.

• *Beta-carotene and other carotenoids.* Found in kale, sweet potatoes, spinach and tomatoes.

• *Bioflavonoids.* Found in blueberries, red grapes, raspberries and beets.

• *Saponins.* Found in soy foods.

Since different phytochemicals boost immunity differently, it's best to eat a variety of fruits and vegetables.

Half the vegetables you eat should be orange or red. Half should be dark green.

Focus on fruits that are colorful all the way through—blueberries, cherries, oranges, etc.

SPICE POWER: Garlic, ginger and turmeric (the main ingredient in curry) have powerful immunity-stimulating effects.

Each day, take three cloves of garlic (or four 500-milligram [mg] garlic pills)...two half-teaspoons of ginger (or four 500-mg ginger pills)...and one-quarter teaspoon of turmeric (or two 500-mg turmeric pills).

EXERCISE AND SLEEP...

Exercise boosts immunity by stimulating the activity of natural killer cells. These specialized white blood cells destroy other cells in the body that have been infected with viruses.

Aim for at least 30 minutes of aerobic activity per day. Walking is less likely to cause injury than running, bicycling and other more vigorous activities.

Like exercise, sleep boosts immunity by enhancing natural killer-cell activity. The average healthy person needs seven to nine hours of sleep per night. During periods of illness, the need for sleep can rise to 10 or even 11 hours per night.

NUTRITIONAL SUPPLEMENTS...

Even the best diet won't give you all the vitamins and minerals needed for strong immune function.

Some nutrients are difficult to get from diet alone, since they occur in foods eaten only rarely. And to counter the growing threat posed by ozone, nitric oxide and other immunity-impairing pollutants, we need more antioxidant vitamins and minerals than our ancestors did.

Ask your doctor about taking flaxseed oil* (one tablespoon or five capsules per day), along with a daily supplement or supplements containing...

- *Folic acid*...800 micrograms (mcg)
- *Vitamin B-6*...10 mg
- *Vitamin C*...500 mg
- *Vitamin D*...400 to 800 international units (IU)
- *Vitamin E*...200 to 400 IU**
- *Chromium*...200 to 400 mcg
- *Copper*...0.5 to 1.0 mg
- *Manganese*...10 to 20 mg
- *Molybdenum*...200 to 400 mcg
- *Selenium*...100 to 200 mcg
- *Zinc*...15 to 20 mg.

TRAP 1: Too much iron interferes with the absorption of certain minerals...and can be dangerous for people with *hemochromatosis,* an iron metabolism disorder that is often undiagnosed. Take supplemental iron only if a doctor tells you to.

TRAP 2: Calcium can interfere with the absorption of trace minerals. If you take a calcium supplement, be sure to take it at least two hours before or after taking your vitamin/mineral pills.

ALCOHOL AND TOBACCO...

If you drink, drink only red wine—it's an excellent source of flavonoids—and limit your consumption to one glass per day. Grape juice contains flavonoids without the alcohol.

*Flaxseed oil contains high levels of alphalinoleic acid, an omega-3 fatty acid that helps regulate immune response. If you prefer, grind one tablespoon of flaxseeds in a clean coffee grinder and add to cereal.

**Due to the possible interactions between vitamin E and various drugs and supplements, as well as other safety considerations, be sure to consult your doctor before starting a vitamin E regimen.

Tobacco in any form decreases immune function by flooding the body with free radicals.

NEEDLESS MEDICATION...

Your stomach and intestines are the first line of defense against food-borne bacteria and parasites.

Because stomach acid kills bacteria, it's a good idea to minimize your use of acid-lowering drugs like *cimetidine* (Tagamet) and *ranitidine* (Zantac)—unless a doctor recommends them.

Antibiotics can decimate the "good" bacteria that live in your gut. That can leave you vulnerable to infection by disease-causing bacteria.

If you must take an antibiotic, ask your doctor about also taking a supplement containing the good bacterium *Lactobacillus plantarium.* It's the only variety not harmed by antibiotics.

HOUSEHOLD MOLD...

Many molds found around the house produce substances toxic to the immune system.

TO CONTROL MOLD: Keep windows open a crack for ventilation...use a dehumidifier...use exhaust fans when showering or cooking...eliminate carpeting in damp rooms...and clean shower stalls and other mold-prone areas with a solution made of equal parts hydrogen peroxide and water.

Keep humidity in your home less than 50%. Test the humidity periodically with a *hygrometer,* an inexpensive instrument sold at hardware stores.

FORMALDEHYDE AND BENZENE...

Formaldehyde—which is sometimes found in clothing, furniture, wall paint, nail polish and hair spray—neutralizes immune cells.

Check labels. Avoid products that contain formaldehyde. Allow new clothes to "off-gas" by airing them in an empty, well-ventilated room for several days.

If possible, allow new carpeting, wall paint and upholstered furniture to off-gas for at least a week before living with them.

NEXT TIME YOU REDECORATE: Use latex wall paint and formaldehyde-free carpeting.

Another ubiquitous compound with immunity-depleting properties is benzene. Found in everything from room deodorizers to gasoline, benzene has a toxic effect on white blood cells.

If you pump your own gasoline, use a pump with a fume-containing nozzle and keep your face turned away.

■

HIP FRACTURES MAY HEAL FASTER WITH PROTEIN

Source: **Marc-André Schürch, MD,** resident, department of internal medicine, University Hospital, Geneva, Switzerland. His six-month study of 82 elderly patients was published in the *Annals of Internal Medicine,* 190 N. Independence Mall W., Philadelphia 19106.

Hip fractures may heal faster when the sufferer boosts protein consumption. In one study, hip fracture patients who took a daily supplement containing 20 grams of milk protein showed less bone loss than similar patients given a placebo. The protein-supplement patients also left the hospital sooner. Hip fracture patients should discuss their protein needs with a doctor or specialist.

■

SOY FOODS CAN HELP YOU AVOID HEART DISEASE, CANCER AND OSTEOPOROSIS

Source: **Mark Messina, PhD,** adjunct associate professor of nutrition at Loma Linda University School of Medicine in Loma Linda, CA. He is coauthor of *The Simple Soybean and Your Health.* Avery.

Can a diet rich in soybeans prevent cancer and heart disease? How about osteoporosis?

In the past few years, a growing chorus of researchers have touted the health benefits of the soybean. An age-old staple of

Asian cuisine, this lowly legume was, until recently, a stranger to American kitchens.

It's not yet clear that soy is the disease-preventing wonder food its proponents say it is, but the research is very promising.

HIGH NUTRITIONAL VALUE...

Like meat and milk, soy is a great source of protein. Unlike these animal proteins, soy is cholesterol-free and low in saturated fat.

Soy also contains dietary fiber and key nutrients like calcium, folate, omega-3 fatty acids and a class of compounds called *isoflavones*.

In addition to weakly mimicking the hormone estrogen, isoflavones act as antioxidants. They guard the body against free radicals—renegade molecules thought to contribute to heart disease, cancer, cataracts and a range of other ailments.

SOY AND HEART DISEASE...

Soy protein and isoflavones work together to prevent heart disease. Study after study has shown that eating 25 grams (g) of soy protein a day—the equivalent of three servings of soy foods—cuts levels of LDL (bad) cholesterol by as much as 10%.

Unlike a low-fat diet—the usual approach to lowering LDL levels—a soy-rich diet does not lower levels of HDL (good) cholesterol. And in women, soy raises levels of HDL cholesterol—thereby reducing the risk for heart disease.

A 10% reduction in LDL isn't quite the 30% to 60% reduction that is possible with cholesterol-lowering drugs. But unlike drugs, soy causes no side effects.

Soy also stops the oxidation of LDL cholesterol. Only oxidized LDL is believed to accumulate on coronary artery walls.

REDUCED RISK FOR CANCER...

It's well known that cancers of the breast, colon and prostate are less prevalent in Japan than in the US. But why? Epidemiologists theorize that the high consumption of soy in Japan may be part of the explanation.

This theory seems to be supported by these findings...

• *Prostate cancer.* The soybean isoflavone *genistein* inhibited the growth of human prostate cancer cells that had been transplanted into rodents.

• *Tumor spread.* The spread of cancer cells through the body—a process known as *metastasis*—was inhibited by soy protein and genistein. Human skin tumors transplanted into rodents were less likely to spread to the lungs among the animals fed soy than among similar animals fed nonsoy feed.

Soy inhibits cancer by curbing cell division, the process that runs amok in cases of cancer. It also seems to inhibit *angiogenesis*—the process by which new blood vessels form to support the growth and spread of tumors.

• *Breast cancer.* Several studies have shown a reduced incidence of breast cancer among lab animals fed soy or a fermented soy product called *miso.*

CAUTION: Some studies have shown that eating lots of soy can actually *promote* the growth of breast cells. In theory, this could mean an increased rather than a decreased risk for breast cancer.

Until more data is in, women with breast cancer should discuss soy consumption with a doctor.

HOT FLASHES AND OSTEOPOROSIS...

Hot flashes and other menopausal symptoms occur when estrogen levels dwindle. Thanks to their estrogen-like properties, isoflavones curb these symptoms—at least in some women.

In an Italian study, women who ate two or three daily servings of soy reported a 45% decrease in hot flashes. A placebo group reported only a 30% decrease.

Numerous studies with rats have shown that the consumption of soy strengthens bones and helps prevent osteoporosis.

There is little research involving humans to corroborate these studies. But two newer studies suggest that soy can retard bone loss in postmenopausal women. Ask your doctor.

ADDING SOY TO YOUR DIET...

Soy comes in many different varieties, all of which are now sold in supermarkets...

• *Tofu.* Also known as bean curd, this nearly tasteless food is a pleasant addition to salads, stir-fries and pasta sauces. One-half cup contains 30 milligrams (mg) of isoflavones and about 10 g of soy protein.

• *Tempeh.* This cooked, fermented product has a meaty texture and a slightly nutty taste. It has roughly the same iso-flavone/protein content as tofu.

• *Soy milk.* It can be used just like cow's milk—as a beverage, poured on cereal, etc. One cup contains 25 mg of isoflavones and about 7 g of soy protein.

Other sources of soy include textured vegetable protein, which can be used instead of meat in sauces, casseroles, etc....and prepared foods like soy burgers, soy hot dogs and soy lasagna.

CAUTION: Soy sauce, soy oil and certain other soy foods contain no isoflavones. If the label doesn't mention isoflavone content, call the manufacturer to find out.

Eat two or three servings of soy-based food each day. If that's too much for you, consider taking a daily isoflavone supplement.

Soy supplements do not contain soy protein and they have not been shown to lower cholesterol.

■

VITAMIN SUPPLEMENTS FIGHT CATARACTS

Source: **M. Cristina Leske, MD, MPH,** distinguished professor, preventive medicine and ophthalmology, School of Medicine, Stony Brook University, Stony Brook,
NY. Her four-year study of 764 men and women was published in *Ophthalmology*,
655 Beach St., San Francisco 94109.

In a study, regular users of multivitamin supplements were one-third less likely than nonusers to develop *nuclear* cataracts—the most common type. Those who took daily vitamin E supplements cut their risk in half. Consult your doctor for the appropriate amount for you.

■

HERBAL REMEDIES: SECRETS OF GREATER EFFECTIVENESS AND SAFER USE

Source: **Ethan Russo, MD,** clinical associate professor of medicine at the University of Washington School of Medicine in Seattle. He is author of *The Handbook of Psychotropic Herbs.* Haworth Press.

People often assume that because herbs are "natural," they pose little risk. Not true.

Some herbs are too toxic for medicinal use. Even some that are generally safe can cause liver or kidney damage.

And like prescription medications, herbal remedies can react dangerously with certain drugs or foods.

How can you use herbal remedies for maximum safety and effectiveness? **DR. ETHAN RUSSO SETS DOWN THESE GUIDELINES...**

• *Avoid herbs known to be dangerous.* Given their inherent dangers, it's best to avoid chaparral, comfrey, life root, germander, coltsfoot, sassafras and ma huang.

• *Don't be misled by wild claims.* Federal law forbids herbal remedy manufacturers from saying their products offer outright cures. But manufacturers often tout their products as providing relief from a ludicrously wide range of ailments.

Take manufacturers' claims with a grain of salt. The best manufacturers often make no health claims for their products.

• *Seek reliable information.* The average doctor knows little about herbs. The same is true for the average druggist.

Health food store clerks may sound knowledgeable, but their information often comes from herbal remedy manufacturers—hardly a source of unbiased information.

The most reliable source of information on herbs is *The Complete German Commission E Monographs: Therapeutic Guide to Herbal Medicines,* American Botanical Council (ABC).* You can contact the ABC by calling 512-926-4900 or going on to its Web site at *www.herbalgram.org.*

• *Work with a knowledgeable practitioner.* For referral to an herb-savvy medical doctor in your area, you can also contact the American Botanical Council.

*Your library may have this book. If not, it can be ordered from the American Botanical Council...or via an online bookseller.

ALTERNATIVE: See a naturopathic physician. In addition to basic medical training, naturopaths have extensive instruction in the safe use of herbs.

• *Buy only standardized formulations.* Standardized herbal extracts have been formulated to provide the active ingredient or ingredients at a specific concentration. That way, you're assured the product is both potent and safe to use.

Look for the word "standardized" or the words "German standards" on the label.

• *Follow label directions carefully.* Like drugs, herbs work best at specific dosages. Take only the recommended dosage, and be sure to take the herb with or without meals, water, etc.—as indicated.

• *Don't mix herbs and drugs.* Herbs can boost the potency of certain medications. If you're taking a prescription drug, don't begin taking any herbal extract until you've checked with a physician or naturopath.

If a doctor has prescribed a drug for you, let him/her know about any herbal remedies you're already taking. He may need to adjust the dosage.

Common herb–drug interactions include...

• *St. John's wort* and *fluoxetine* (Prozac). The combination can raise brain levels of the neurotransmitter serotonin. "Serotonin syndrome" can cause delirium and other symptoms.

• *Ginkgo biloba* and anticoagulants. Like aspirin, *warfarin* (Coumadin) and other anticoagulants, ginkgo thins the blood. Taken along with an anticoagulant, ginkgo can inhibit proper clotting and cause internal bleeding.

• *Watch out for allergic reactions.* Introduce herbs one at a time. Don't add a second herb until you've taken the first for an entire week without experiencing any symptoms of an allergic reaction, such as rash, upset stomach, dizziness or headache.

If you experience any of these symptoms, stop taking the herb at once. Try taking it again one week later. If symptoms return, stop taking the herb for good.

CAUTION: If you become short of breath after taking an herb, call for an ambulance at once.

• *Don't take herbs during pregnancy.* Ginger, garlic and other herbs that are popular as foods are generally okay. But other herbs can cause serious problems for pregnant women.

It's also best to check with a doctor before giving any herbal remedy to a child under age 12.

■

GARLIC AND YOUR HEALTH

Source: **John Milner, PhD,** professor and head of the department of nutrition at Pennsylvania State University in University Park. Dr. Milner chaired a major conference on the health benefits of garlic.

S tudies conducted in the US, Europe and China suggest that garlic can lower cholesterol levels...fight bacterial and viral infections...prevent cancer...and boost memory.

How strong is the evidence? Could you benefit by adding more garlic to your diet...or by taking garlic pills?

GARLIC VS. CHOLESTEROL...

As proponents of garlic are quick to point out, numerous studies suggest that regular consumption of garlic—one clove a day or the equivalent in supplement form—cuts serum cholesterol by 7% to 15%. Garlic seems to be especially helpful at reducing LDL (bad) cholesterol.

Other studies suggest that garlic has little or no effect on cholesterol levels.

EXAMPLE: A study conducted at the University of Bonn and published in the *Journal of the American Medical Association* showed that cholesterol levels remained unchanged even when garlic oil equivalent to four to five cloves of garlic was consumed on a daily basis for 12 weeks.

What explains the inconsistency of the studies? It may be that only some people respond to garlic. It's also possible that garlic interacts with the other foods in one's diet.

Another possible explanation for the inconsistency may be the fact that the studies have used various garlic preparations. Some have used unprocessed garlic. Others have used a garlic extract—which might or might not have the same biological activity as whole garlic.

GARLIC VS. CANCER...

Research suggests that garlic can help prevent a variety of common malignancies...

• *Stomach cancer.* In a study conducted in China, people who ate garlic regularly had an unusually low rate of this potentially deadly cancer.

• *Colon cancer.* A study of women in Iowa found that the incidence of colon cancer was 50% lower among those who consumed the most garlic.

• *Prostate cancer.* A study conducted in Oxford, England, found that men who consumed garlic two or more times per week were one-third less likely than other men to develop prostate cancer.

If garlic does protect against cancer, the explanation may lie in the sulfur compounds it contains.

Some laboratory studies have demonstrated that these compounds block the synthesis of carcinogens known as *nitrosamines.* In the absence of sulfur, the digestive process leads to the formation of nitrosamines each time nitrates and nitrites are consumed.

Nitrates and nitrites are found in preservatives and in beets, spinach and certain other foods.

Garlic also stimulates the body to synthesize *glutathione.* In addition to deactivating certain carcinogens, this natural antioxidant protects cell membranes against damage caused by renegade molecules known as free radicals.

Recent studies suggest that it might be possible to derive cancer chemotherapy drugs from garlic.

In one recent study, a garlic derivative called *S-allylmercaptocysteine* inhibited the growth of human prostate tumors that had been transplanted to mice.

In another study, a garlic extract called *diallyldisulfide* inhibited the growth of human breast cancer cells.

HOW TO EAT GARLIC...

There is no *proof* that garlic can reduce cholesterol, lower cancer risk or do anything else to protect your health. But given the evidence in garlic's favor—plus the fact that the only universal downside is bad breath—it makes sense to include some in your diet unless you have an allergy.

One to three grams of garlic per day—the equivalent of one clove—should be enough.

If you cook with garlic, be careful to preserve the potentially beneficial sulfur compounds. To do this, peel garlic, chop or crush it and then let it stand for 15 to 30 minutes before cooking. This "waiting period" facilitates chemical reactions that yield the biologically active compounds.

If you don't like the taste or smell of garlic, deodorized supplements are available. These products contain compounds similar to those found in raw garlic.

■

MULTIVITAMINS CAN BOOST IMMUNITY

Source: **John Bogden, PhD, MS,** professor of preventive medicine and community health, New Jersey Medical School, Newark.

Multivitamins significantly boosted immunity in people age 60 or older. Researchers found a 60% improvement in immune responses in seniors who took a multivitamin supplement daily for a year, but no significant change in those given placebos. The results suggest that older people benefit from higher levels of vitamins and minerals than the recommended daily allowance (RDA).

■

CANCER FIGHTERS

CANCER SELF-DEFENSE: SIMPLE METHOD

Source: **Edward L. Giovannucci, MD,** professor of nutrition and epidemiology, Harvard School of Public Health, Boston. The 20-year study of 121,701 nurses was published in *The New England Journal of Medicine,* 10 Shattuck St., Boston 02115.

Aspirin may *halve* colon cancer risk. It has long been thought that aspirin reduces the risk of colon and rectal cancer, but researchers have never been able to pinpoint how much and how often aspirin should be taken to achieve the greatest benefits.

A study found that female nurses who took as few as four to six aspirin a week lowered their risks of colon and rectal cancer by 44%.

HOWEVER: These benefits didn't accrue until the women had been taking the aspirin for at least a decade.

THEORY: Aspirin may have an effect only on the earliest stages of the disease, by preventing the formation of polyps that might develop into cancerous tumors years later. An aspirin a day or every second day may be sufficient to reduce the risk of colon cancer. See your physician before starting this program.

■

OVER-THE-COUNTER CANCER FIGHTER

Source: **Daniel W. Cramer, MD**, professor of obstetrics and gynecology, Brigham and Women's Hospital, Boston. His study of over-the-counter painkiller use among 1,086 women was published in *The Lancet,* 32 Jamestown Rd., London NW1 7BY.

Ovarian cancer risk may be lowered via regular use of *acetaminophen* (Tylenol). In a preliminary study, women who used acetaminophen once a day were 61% less likely than other women to develop ovarian cancer. Further research is needed to confirm this finding.

KNOWN RISK REDUCERS: Taking oral contraceptives and avoiding talc. Women with a family history of ovarian cancer should consider being tested for the genes associated with the disease. Ask your doctor.

■

THE MAGNIFICENT ANTICANCER MARINADE

Do you like to barbecue? If so, you may have heard that grilled meats often contain high levels of carcinogenic compounds called *heterocyclic amines* (HCAs).

This special marinade—developed by molecular biologist James Felton, PhD, and his colleagues at Lawrence Livermore National Laboratory in Livermore, California—keeps the formation of HCAs to a minimum.

The researchers aren't quite certain exactly *how* it works —only that it does. The marinade is especially effective when used with chicken, although it works with other meats as well.

The following is enough for one chicken.

6 tablespoons olive oil
4 tablespoons cider vinegar

4 tablespoons lemon juice
½ cup packed brown sugar
3 tablespoons grainy mustard
3 medium garlic cloves, crushed
1½ teaspoons salt

Mix all ingredients together in a bowl. Place the meat and enough marinade to cover it in a resealable plastic bag. Soak for four hours, making sure the meat remains covered.

■

IMPORTANT BREAKTHROUGHS IN CANCER CARE

Source: The late **Gerald P. Murphy, MD,** former director of research at the Pacific Northwest Cancer Foundation and Northwest Hospital in Seattle and former chief medical officer of the American Cancer Society.

Had cancer researchers at last found a cure for cancer? That tantalizing possibility was raised by a *New York Times* article that described an experimental therapy developed by the late Dr. Judah Folkman, a researcher at Children's Hospital in Boston.

Folkman had cured cancer in lab mice using the experimental drugs *endostatin* and *angiostatin.*

Excitement over this news soon ebbed. While Folkman's work is promising, follow-up stories pointed out that the drugs might not work in humans.

Even if the drugs do work in humans, it could be years before they receive Food and Drug Administration (FDA) approval.

GOOD NEWS: Anti-angiogenesis therapy is just one of many breakthroughs in cancer therapy. **MANY OTHER BREAKTHROUGHS ARE AVAILABLE RIGHT NOW...**

CONFORMAL RADIATION...

With conventional radiation therapy, doctors know only the position of the tumor they're bombarding with radiation.

Since they don't know the tumor's shape, it's hard for them to limit the delivery of radiation only to the cancerous tissue. Some radiation inevitably "spills over" onto healthy tissue.

With conformal radiation therapy, doctors use three-dimensional imaging technology to plot the tumor's shape and position. That way, high doses of radiation can be delivered accurately and with minimal damage to the surrounding healthy tissue.

GAMMA KNIFE...

Used to treat brain tumors, this noninvasive tool can focus radiation with surgical precision.

The gamma knife is less risky than conventional surgery or radiation therapy. Brain tumors can be removed with little or no damage to surrounding tissue.

Recovery time is faster, too. In most cases, the treatment lasts less than one hour and the patient goes home the next day.

Conventional brain surgery typically requires at least three days in the hospital and four to six weeks of at-home recovery.

LYMPHATIC MAPPING...

With cancers that spread through the lymphatic system, such as breast cancer, surgeons used to remove not only the cancerous organ but also most or all of the lymph nodes under the armpit. This can lead to *lymphedema,* a painful and disfiguring swelling of the arm. It can also leave the arm highly vulnerable to infection.

Lymphatic mapping helps prevent lymphedema by limiting the number of lymph nodes removed.

After the tumor is cut out—while the patient is still on the operating table—dye is injected near the tumor site.

By noting where the dye drains into the lymphatic system, the surgeon can pinpoint which lymph nodes should be removed and examined for cancer. That permits less extensive surgery.

RADIOACTIVE SEEDING...

With conventional radiation therapy, radiation from a machine is beamed at the tumor. But researchers have found that radiation can be delivered more effectively to certain tumors by seeding them with tiny radioactive pellets.

The pellets deliver radiation to cancerous tissue without damaging nearby healthy cells.

Known as *brachytherapy*, this seeding technique has proven effective for cancers of the prostate and pancreas.

Used against prostate cancer, brachytherapy has proven just as effective as conventional radiation therapy and surgery —with a smaller risk for impotence or incontinence.

MONOCLONAL ANTIBODIES...

Chemotherapy is often highly effective at killing cancer cells. But since the drugs used in chemotherapy affect healthy cells as well as cancerous ones, patients undergoing chemotherapy often experience toxic reactions, such as impaired heart, liver or kidney function.

Using gene-splicing technology, researchers have been able to clone cancer-killing antibodies directly from the cells of cancer patients. These monoclonal antibody drugs attack cancer cells—but leave healthy cells alone.

The first monoclonal antibody drug to hit the market, *rituximab* (Rituxan), was approved by the FDA in 1997. It has proven highly effective against non-Hodgkin's lymphoma.

Trastuzumab (Herceptin), a genetically engineered monoclonal antibody, has proven effective in slowing the progression of advanced breast cancer. Herceptin is currently being tested on earlier-stage breast cancer to see if it can delay or prevent the spread of the disease, as well as on some cases of ovarian and prostate cancer.

FINDING GOOD CANCER CARE...

How can cancer patients be sure that they're receiving state-of-the-art care? One way is to be treated at a facility funded by the National Cancer Institute (NCI). To find out if there's one near you, call the NCI at 800-422-6237 or look on the Web at *www.nci.nih.gov*. You can also contact them to learn about treatment options and clinical trials.

First-rate cancer care is also available at institutions accredited by the American College of Surgeons (ACS).

To find an accredited facility near you, check the Web site *www.facs.org*—or call the ACS at 312-202-5085.

■

SKIN CANCER ALERT

Source: **Henry S. Kahn, MD,** professor emeritus of family and preventive medicine, Emory University School of Medicine, Atlanta.

Melanoma isn't the only form of skin cancer that can have serious consequences.

FINDING: Having had *non*melanoma skin cancer (basal cell or squamous cell carcinoma) raises by roughly 25% the risk of dying from serious malignancies, including melanoma, lymphoma, leukemia and cancers of the salivary glands, pharynx, breast, lung and prostate. Patients with nonmelanoma skin cancer should be monitored carefully by their doctors.

■

CANCER SURGERY FOR ELDERLY PATIENTS

Source: **Garrett Walsh, MD,** professor of thoracic and cardiovascular surgery, University of Texas M.D. Anderson Cancer Center, Houston. His 13-year study of 1,400 cancer operations was presented at a meeting of the Royal College of Physicians and Surgeons.

Cancer surgery should be an option even for elderly patients.

TRAP: Doctors often consider patients age 70 or older too old to withstand surgery.

FINDING: Older lung cancer patients who underwent surgery were no more likely to experience complications or die as a result of surgery than were younger patients with similar problems.

BOTTOM LINE: Age alone should not preclude a patient from undergoing cancer surgery.

■

HEALTHIER
HEARTS

POTASSIUM PILLS LOWER
HIGH BLOOD PRESSURE

Source: **Frank M. Sacks, MD,** professor of cardiovascular disease prevention, Harvard School of Public Health, Boston. His study of blood pressure in 300 women was published in *Hypertension,* University of Mississippi Medical Center, 2500 N. State St., Jackson, MS, 39216.

Potassium pills work better than calcium or magnesium pills at lowering blood pressure. In a study of people with normal blood pressure, a daily pill containing 1,600 milligrams (mg) of potassium lowered systolic pressure (the top number) by two points and diastolic pressure (the bottom number) by 1.7 points. Even such slight reductions cut the risk for stroke and heart attack. Researchers theorize that potassium's pressure-lowering effect is greater in people with high blood pressure. If you have high blood pressure, ask your doctor about taking potassium supplements.

■

VITAMIN E VS. HEART ATTACKS

Source: **Howard N. Hodis, MD,** director of the atherosclerosis research unit, Keck School of Medicine, University of Southern California, Los Angeles.

Heart attacks were cut by 40% in nurses who took vitamin E supplements. In another study, examination of the arteries of men who had undergone bypass surgery found that lesions related to heart disease were smaller after they had taken vitamin E for two years. Scientists believe the positive effect is probably due to the vitamin's antioxidant properties.

CAUTION: More than 200 IU can be dangerous. Consult your doctor for the amount that is appropriate for you.

■

VITAMIN D VS. HIGH BLOOD PRESSURE

Source: **Betty Drees, MD,** dean, University of Missouri at Kansas City School of Medicine.

Too little vitamin D may contribute to high blood pressure. A 10-year study of patients 40 to 60 years of age showed a relationship between low blood levels of vitamin D and higher blood pressures.

SELF-DEFENSE: Each day, consume 400 international units (IU) of vitamin D. One cup of milk contains 100 IU.

OTHER SOURCES: Cod liver oil, mackerel, salmon, sardines and fortified breakfast cereals.

■

SOLUTIONS TO COMMON PROBLEMS

12 THINGS YOU CAN DO IN UNDER FIVE MINUTES EACH TO IMPROVE YOUR HEALTH

Source: **Harold H. Bloomfield, MD,** psychiatrist in private practice in Del Mar, CA. He is coauthor of *The Power of 5*. Rodale Press.

We'd all like to lead healthier, happier lives. But many of us feel so pressed for time that we fail to take the steps required to make that happen.

No more excuses. Here are ways to boost your health and happiness—*in five minutes or less.*

1. *Inhale an energizing scent.* Research suggests that lemon and peppermint scents are energizing. To exploit this finding, have an occasional cup of lemon or peppermint tea...or chew peppermint gum. Keep a bottle of peppermint and/or lemon extract to sniff...add a couple of drops to a small scent dispenser...or experiment with potpourri containing other energizing scents such as pine, jasmine, lavender, orange or grapefruit.

2. *Sip ice water.* It keeps your cells hydrated *and* helps you burn calories. *Reason:* Whenever you drink something cold, your body raises your metabolism to keep your body temperature from falling. That process burns calories—eight 16-ounce glasses of ice water will burn an extra 200 calories per day.

STRATEGY: Start the day with eight to 16 ounces of ice water. Sip a 16-ounce glass every hour or two, keeping one next to you at work and at home. All told, you should drink eight glasses a day. Finish up by 7 pm—to avoid having to use the bathroom after you go to bed.

3. *Practice "one-breath" meditation.* You don't have to spend years mastering meditation. This one-breath method is a powerful, straightforward relaxation technique that can be practiced anytime, anywhere. Try it whenever you feel fatigued or out of sorts.

WHAT TO DO: Sit in a comfortable chair. Straighten your back, relax your shoulders and take a deep breath. Let the air "open" your chest. Imagine it filling every cell in your body. Hold the breath for a moment, then exhale, releasing every bit of tension.

ALSO HELPFUL: One-touch relaxation. Place your fingertips just in front of your ears. Inhale and clench your teeth. Hold for five seconds. Exhale, and let your jaw muscles go loose.

Repeat this exercise three more times, using half the original tension, then one-fourth, then one-eighth. Then take a deep breath, press your fingertips against your jaw, let it go slack and say, *Ah-h-h-h.* Imagine you are breathing out tightness.

4. *Minimize noise at home and at work.* Loud or irritating sound creates severe emotional and physical tension. Fortunately, many aggravating noises can be silenced.

STRATEGY 1: Place foam pads under blenders and other kitchen appliances...and under printers and other office machines.

STRATEGY 2: Before buying an air conditioner or another potentially noisy appliance, compare noise levels of different brands. Use noise-absorbing insulation around dishwashers.

5. *Bask in bright light.* Most people get a powerful surge of energy from sunlight or bright indoor light. Make use of this effect by moving your desk chair closer to a window...or take a five-minute outdoor walk every few hours.

ALSO HELPFUL: Each day, get five minutes of nonpeak sun (before 10 am or after 3 pm) without sunscreen or sunglasses to enjoy the full mood-lifting effects of sunlight.

Indoors, replace incandescent or fluorescent bulbs with full-spectrum "daylight" bulbs available at lighting or health food stores.

6. Do abdominal exercises. Use this technique while sitting at your desk or while stuck in traffic. Sit up straight. Place hands on hips with thumbs pointing toward your back. Exhale slowly and completely, pushing the last air out forcefully with your lower abdominals.

Repeat up to 10 times a day. You might try one or two stomach-flattening sessions just before meals, at stoplights on your commute or each time you sit down at your desk. These exercises are great muscle toners for the lower abdomen.

7. Perform mental "cross-training." Cross-training is the process by which you "stretch" your mind in as many different directions as possible by engaging in a variety of mental and physical activities. Word puzzles and other games are an easy way to perform this cross-training. Pick a random sentence from the newspaper, then rearrange the words to make a new sentence...play *Scrabble* or do crossword puzzles...challenge a friend to chess, checkers or bridge.

8. Cook with "nutriceuticals." These are vegetables, herbs and spices that have specific healing properties...

• Garlic and onions boost the immune system, helping prevent colds.

• Basil, cumin and turmeric help prevent cancer of the bladder and prostate.

• Black pepper, jalapeños, mustard and hot red peppers all boost your metabolism for several hours. That helps burn fat.

• Cinnamon helps metabolize sugar, keeping your blood sugar levels steady.

9. Check your reading posture. Poor posture—leaning over a desk, for instance—can cause tension headaches, vision problems and pain in the jaw and/or neck.

SELF-DEFENSE: Bring reading material up to your field of vision or use a book stand to hold a book at the proper angle. If you spend a lot of time on the telephone, get a headset. Don't cradle the phone between ear and shoulder.

10. *Do trigger-point therapy.* Wherever you feel tense, feel for a tight band of muscle tissue—a trigger point. Press or squeeze it with light to moderate pressure. Continue pressing for five to 10 seconds, then release.

11. *Curb indoor pollution.* Whenever possible, keep your windows open. Keep gas appliances properly maintained to limit their output of carbon monoxide. Use exhaust fans in the bathroom, kitchen and garage whenever you use these rooms. All gas appliances should be checked annually—and properly vented to the outside. Make your home and office smoke-free.

12. *Do absolutely nothing.* "Lyming" is the Caribbean art of doing nothing—without feeling guilty about it. Try lyming frequently to give your brain time to process all the information it receives over the course of a day.

HELPFUL: Take a five-minute "mental vacation" every few hours. Picture your favorite beach or other getaway place. The idea is to escape the rat race briefly—but *completely.*

■

CONTROLLING ANXIETY WITHOUT ANTIANXIETY DRUGS

Source: **Harold H. Bloomfield, MD,** psychiatrist in private practice in Del Mar, CA. He is author of more than a dozen books, including *Healing Anxiety Naturally.* HarperPerennial.

Each year, millions of Americans reach for a prescription medication to curb feelings of anxiety. Unfortunately, the *benzodiazepine* tranquilizers doctors often prescribe can cause foggy thinking, memory loss and sleep disturbance...and are highly addictive.

Daily exercise and a low-fat, nutrient-dense diet help fortify the body against the effects of stress. If these measures fail to keep anxiety in check, ask your doctor about herbal remedies.

ST. JOHN'S WORT...

For individuals whose emotional state alternates between anxiety and depression, St. John's wort *(Hypericum perforatum)* is often a good choice.

This herb has proven to be just as effective as prescription antidepressants against mild to moderate depression. Since depression and anxiety often go hand in hand, the herb is widely recommended for anxiety—and for sleep disorders, too.

But you must be patient. The antianxiety effect can take four to six weeks to kick in.

CAUTION: Do *not* take St. John's wort within four weeks of taking a monoamine oxidase (MAO) inhibitor antidepressant, such as *phenelzine* (Nardil) or *tranylcypromine* (Parnate). This combination can trigger a dangerous rise in blood pressure, along with severe anxiety, fever, muscle tension and confusion.

Most studies of St. John's wort extract have involved dosages of 300 milligrams (mg) three times per day. At this level, side effects are mild.

St. John's wort does make the skin more sensitive to sunlight. People with fair skin should use extra sun protection, and those prone to cataracts should wear wraparound sunglasses.

VALERIAN...

Valerian is often helpful when chronic anxiety interferes with the ability to fall asleep or sleep through the night.

Like *triazolam* (Halcion) and other popular sleeping pills, valerian reduces the length of time it takes to fall asleep. Unlike these drugs, valerian produces an entirely "natural" sleep... and is nonaddictive.

The typical dosage of valerian is 900 mg taken one hour before bedtime. If you have chronic insomnia, valerian can take up to two weeks to provide relief.

■

ANTIBALDNESS PILL

Source: **David Freeman,** former editorial director, *Bottom Line/Health,* Boardroom Inc., 281 Tresser Blvd., Stamford, CT 06901.

Even as a man with thinning hair, I didn't give it much thought when the antibaldness pill, *Propecia,* won Food and Drug Administration (FDA) approval. Hair loss affects half of all men. It's not some freakish condition that needs fixing, right?

IN CASE YOU DISAGREE, I PUT A FEW QUESTIONS TO PETER PANAGOTACOS, MD, A HAIR LOSS EXPERT IN SAN FRANCISCO...

• *How effective is Propecia?* Very effective at preventing hair loss, less effective at regrowing lost hair. One-third of Propecia users notice significant hair regrowth, one-third notice some regrowth and one-third notice no regrowth.

Propecia works by blocking the synthesis of the follicle-killing hormone *dihydrotestosterone* (DHT).

• *What about side effects?* Proscar, a higher-dose version of Propecia, has been used for 11 years with no real problems. Propecia should also be safe. The only meaningful side effects —impotence and reduced libido—occur in only a tiny number of Propecia users.

Since prostate trouble is unknown in men whose bodies don't make DHT, some doctors now prescribe Propecia as a way to prevent prostate cancer and/or prostate enlargement.

• *Who should consider taking Propecia?* Any man bothered by hair loss. Given its promise as a prostate protector, Propecia may also be appropriate for men with a family history of prostate trouble.

■

THE GREAT HORMONE DEBATE

Sources: **Christiane Northrup, MD,** physician in private practice in Yarmouth, ME, and former clinical assistant professor of obstetrics and gynecology at the University of Vermont College of Medicine at Maine Medical Center, Portland. She is author of *The Wisdom of Menopause.* Bantam Doubleday Dell...**Joyce Kakkis, MD,** associate professor of obstetrics and gynecology at the University of California-Irvine. She is in private practice in Long Beach, CA, specializing in HRT, and is author of *Confessions of an Estrogen Evangelist.* Kensington.

Doctors have long recommended hormone replacement therapy (HRT) to not only prevent hot flashes and other menopausal symptoms, but also to curb the risk for heart disease and osteoporosis.

But when researchers halted a major study examining the benefits of HRT, millions of women were forced to re-evaluate their options for controlling menopausal symptoms.

After five years of study, researchers conducting the Women's Health Initiative (WHI) found that women who took a daily tablet of synthetic estrogen and synthetic progesterone had a 26% higher rate of breast cancer, a 29% higher rate of heart attack and a 41% higher rate of stroke than those taking a placebo. As a result of these findings, the 16,808 women being studied were instructed to stop taking the medications—immediately.

Is this the last word on HRT? For answers, we interviewed two leading experts in women's health—physicians who have addressed these questions for themselves and for their patients.

Christiane Northrup, MD, is menopausal (complete cessation of periods) and favors the use of natural treatments for menopausal symptoms.

Joyce Kakkis, MD, is perimenopausal (the years preceding menopause, when periods become irregular) and favors the use of HRT.

DR. NORTHRUP...

What is your opinion of the WHI study?

I felt that the study had major flaws from the outset. Women took a pill consisting of estrogen made from the urine of a pregnant mare, in combination with a chemically synthesized form of the hormone progesterone.

In all the years of human evolution, except for about the last 50, these chemicals have never been introduced into human bodies. And this so-called medicine—prescribed at the same dosage for millions of women, whether they weighed 110 or 210 pounds—was supposed to reduce the risk for heart disease, osteoporosis and other chronic degenerative diseases. Given that the hormone dosages weren't individualized and didn't match those found in human females, I'm not surprised that there were adverse consequences.

Do you ever recommend HRT?

Yes. Some perimenopausal and menopausal women need hormones to control symptoms or feel their best. Working with her doctor, a woman should have her hormone levels checked and then decide what she needs. Some women's bodies, like mine, make adequate levels of hormones. Others don't. Some women feel best on HRT, while others don't. Women who have had their ovaries removed often need HRT for a few years.

If hormones are recommended, they should be *bio-identical.* This means they are chemically identical to the hormones manufactured in a woman's body, not patented animal versions or synthetic substitutes, which are so widely used today. And the doctor should check hormone levels every year, since a woman's body changes.

What do you use in place of HRT?

Soy does nearly everything HRT does without any of the side effects. I use soy to help control symptoms, such as hot flashes. Soy can also help control insomnia, dry skin and hair, depression and vaginal dryness, as well as strengthen the bones and heart.

The active ingredient in soy is *isoflavones,* a plant-derived "phytoestrogen" that acts like the estrogen found in the body. Do *not* take isolated soy isoflavones in pill form. Recent studies have shown that large amounts may increase breast cancer risk. Eat soy foods, including edamame (soybeans), soy milk, soy burgers and tofu.

DR. KAKKIS...

What is your opinion of the WHI study?

I think the negative results of the WHI were overstated. By analyzing 10,000 of the study subjects on HRT, researchers found that eight additional women developed breast cancer or had a stroke and seven additional women developed heart disease each year, compared with those not taking HRT.

In light of these findings, should *everyone* stop HRT? I don't think so. Also, most experts think that women who get breast cancer within 10 years of starting HRT have a preexisting condition that was simply accelerated by HRT. In other words, HRT is not the cause of their cancer.

The study also showed some benefits of HRT. Among the women analyzed, six fewer developed colorectal cancer and five fewer suffered hip fracture each year. Should women with a family history of colon cancer and osteoporosis stop HRT? I don't think so.

Finally, quality-of-life issues—hot flashes, insomnia, irritability and depression—were not addressed by this study. I do not intend to stop taking hormones on the basis of the WHI results, nor am I advising my patients to stop.

What's the best way to take HRT?

By using the lowest effective dose, which minimizes the risks. Typically, I start my patients at 25% to 50% of the standard dose of HRT. Then I monitor symptoms every six weeks and gradually increase the dosage only if the lower level is not working. The therapy is individually designed for each woman.

Have your doctor perform blood tests to determine your hormone levels. Then, you should be reevaluated to see whether the therapy is working and to have it adjusted if it is not.

What do you take?

I take birth control pills to control my perimenopausal symptoms. I'm still fertile, so the Pill acts as a contraceptive while providing the needed mix of hormones to prevent the hormonal fluctuations of a perimenopausal woman my age. I intend to go from the Pill to low-dose HRT, and to take it for the rest of my life.

Do you use any natural remedies?

I eat edamame. It makes a delicious dish after 10 minutes of steaming. I have three, one-cup servings a week to control my perimenopausal symptoms.

I also take vitamin E to help control hot flashes and I take calcium to reduce muscle cramps, stabilize my mood and strengthen my bones. Consult your doctor for dosages that are appropriate for you.

■

HOW TO PROTECT YOUR JOINTS FROM OSTEOARTHRITIS

Source: **Doyt Conn, MD,** senior vice president for medical affairs at the Arthritis Foundation, 1330 W. Peachtree St., Atlanta 30309. Contact the foundation at 800-283-7800 or on the Web at *www.arthritis.org* for more on arthritis and for referral to self-help classes in your area.

O steoarthritis is caused by the breakdown of cartilage, the rubbery substance that cushions the joints.

The pain can range from a minor annoyance to a disabling torment. As cartilage slowly wears away, joints become swollen and inflamed. Range of motion often becomes limited.

Knees and hips are the most common sites for osteoarthritis. The lower back, neck, big toe, base of the thumb and finger joints are frequent targets, too.

GOOD NEWS: There are ways to prevent osteoarthritis... and ways to stay active and largely pain-free if you already have the disease.

WHO GETS ARTHRITIS—AND WHY...

Heredity plays a key role in determining who develops osteoarthritis.

Some people have inherited cartilage that is unusually susceptible to wear. Others have inherited low levels of the enzymes that block the inflammatory process underlying cartilage damage.

People who have inherited loose joints, knock knees or bowleggedness are unusually prone to cartilage erosion. The misalignment of their limbs causes their joints to move in ways that increase cartilage wear.

There's not much you can do about heredity or limb alignment, of course. **BUT SEVERAL OTHER OSTEOARTHRITIS RISK FACTORS CAN BE CONTROLLED...**

• *Obesity.* The more you weigh, the greater the burden on your joints.

GOOD NEWS: Losing even a little weight can have a big payoff. In a study of obese women, a loss of just 12 pounds reduced the risk for knee arthritis by 50%.

• *Poor nutrition.* Insufficient intake of vitamin C and/or vitamin D can hasten the progression of osteoarthritis.

Good sources of vitamin C include citrus fruits like oranges and grapefruits, red peppers, tomatoes and strawberries. Vitamin D is found in fortified milk...and is produced by the skin upon exposure to sunlight.

BEWARE: Older people absorb vitamins inefficiently. If you are over age 60, ask your doctor about taking a daily supplement containing 60 milligrams (mg) of vitamin C and 200 international units (IU) of vitamin D.

• *Lack of exercise.* In healthy joints, bone, cartilage and muscle tissue work together to absorb mechanical stresses.

If the muscle around a joint is weakened from disuse, the cartilage and bone must bear all the stress. That subjects the cartilage to greater wear.

SELF-DEFENSE: Get regular exercise. Exercise helps build the muscles that provide extra support to vulnerable joints. It also stimulates the growth of new cartilage. In addition to walking, bicycling and swimming, consider strength training for your lower body.

• *Having a "trick" joint.* Joints that have been injured—or operated upon—tend to age more rapidly than healthy joints.

SELF-DEFENSE: If you have a bad knee or another problem joint, use caution when exercising. Walking or bicycling subjects the knee to less stress than running.

ARTHRITIS TREATMENTS...

People with osteoarthritis often benefit from heating pads and cold compresses...and from specialized exercises that target the muscle attached to the painful joint.

FOR OSTEOARTHRITIS OF THE KNEE: Lie on your back on the floor, with your right leg bent and right foot flat on the floor. Extend your left leg. Raise your left leg off the floor six inches. Hold for a count of 10 before lowering your leg. Repeat 12 times. Switch legs and repeat.

FOR OSTEOARTHRITIS OF THE BACK: Lie on your back on the floor, with your knees bent and feet flat on the floor. Flatten your back against the floor by tightening your buttocks and stomach muscles. Raise your head and shoulders as high as is comfortably possible. Hold for a count of three. Lower. Repeat eight times.

If exercise and heat or cold fail to control the pain, medication often helps. Acetaminophen is usually the first choice. Ibuprofen, naproxen and other nonsteroidal anti-inflammatory drugs (NSAIDs) can be more effective when arthritic joints are swollen and inflamed.

CAUTION: NSAIDs should be used on a daily basis for no longer than three weeks—because of the risk of stomach irritation and other side effects. If you have a history of ulcers or stomach trouble, consult a doctor before trying NSAIDs.

For pain that cannot be relieved with oral medication, an injection of a cortisone derivative such as *betamethasone* (Celestone) often helps.

Another option is an injection of *hyaluronic acid* (HA). A single injection of this natural joint-lubricating compound can lessen pain for months.

Joint replacement surgery is usually reserved for cases involving severe, disabling pain that cannot be controlled by medication or other measures.

The operation takes about two hours, with a total hospital stay of roughly one week, followed by a two-month convalescence at home.

WHAT ABOUT SUPPLEMENTS?...

In recent years, the media have been filled with reports of arthritis sufferers who experienced dramatic pain relief after taking *glucosamine* and *chondroitin sulfate*.

Studies show that glucosamine controls pain as well as NSAIDs. But there is no proof that either supplement repairs cartilage.

CAUTION: These supplements are poorly regulated by the Food and Drug Administration (FDA), so it's hard to know how pure any given product is.

An arthritis remedy called NutraJoint is said to help maintain cartilage health by providing the body with gelatin, vitamin C and calcium.

Reports suggest that people who take NutraJoint on a daily basis experience pain relief.

■

AMAZING WAYS TO CONTROL RHEUMATOID ARTHRITIS

Source: **James F. Fries, MD,** professor of medicine and rheumatology at Stanford University School of Medicine in Stanford, CA. He is coauthor of *The Arthritis Helpbook.* Da Capo Press.

If you're among the estimated two million Americans who have rheumatoid arthritis (RA), there's good news.

Current treatment strategies are proving to be much more effective than the strategies that were considered state of the art just a short time ago.

IMPLICATION: If you have RA but haven't seen a doctor recently, your current treatment regimen may not be optimal.

An autoimmune disease, RA occurs when the immune system attacks the body's own cells as if they were invaders.

This attack causes the joints to become swollen and warm to the touch. Enzymes produced in the joints as a result of this inflammation slowly digest adjacent tissue, causing permanent damage to bone and cartilage.

Joint damage begins earlier in the disease process than many RA patients—and even some doctors—realize. For this reason, it's crucial that treatment be initiated without delay.

IMPORTANT: Consult a rheumatologist. Given all the recent advances, few primary care physicians are up-to-date on rheumatoid arthritis treatments.

DRUG SEQUENCING...

The most important advance in the treatment of RA has been the way medications are "sequenced." Traditionally, doctors prescribed potent *disease-modifying antirheumatic drugs* (DMARDs) only after nonsteroidal anti-inflammatory drugs (NSAIDs) proved ineffective.

CURRENT THINKING: It's more effective to prescribe DMARDs first. Doing so ensures that the disease is brought under control as quickly as possible.

Research indicates that *naproxen* (Naprosyn), *ibuprofen* (Advil) and other NSAIDs cause gastrointestinal problems and other serious side effects that are responsible for more than 16,000 deaths and 100,000 hospitalizations each year.

Methotrexate (Rheumatrex), *hydroxychloroquine* (Plaquenil) and other DMARDs now appear to be no riskier than NSAIDs, and are more effective.

BOTTOM LINE: Virtually every rheumatoid arthritis patient should be taking a DMARD. With early and consistent use of DMARDs, lifetime disability can be cut by up to two-thirds.

COMPLETE PAIN RELIEF...

The old approach to treating RA was simply to keep pain levels tolerable.

But since pain stems from tissue damage, even mild discomfort means the disease process is continuing.

BETTER: Treat the disease until pain and stiffness disappear. Speak up if you feel pain. Don't put up with it...and don't assume that it is normal.

Becoming pain-free may take time. Some drugs take up to six weeks to work.

If one DMARD doesn't work, the doctor may try another...or may try a combination of drugs.

MEDICATIONS...

If older, established DMARDs don't work—or if they cause severe side effects—you may be a candidate for one of the newer medications.

The following medications have been approved by the Food and Drug Administration (FDA) for the treatment of rheumatoid arthritis...

• *Leflunomide* (Arava) slows the rate of cell division, inhibiting the reproduction of joint-damaging inflammatory cells. It's often a good option for people who cannot tolerate methotrexate, which can cause mouth ulcers, liver problems and other side effects.

• *Etanercept* (Enbrel) and *infliximab* (Remicade) work by blocking *tumor necrosis factor* (TNF), a naturally occurring compound that activates the inflammatory response.

THE ROLE OF EXERCISE...

Exercise cannot cure RA, but it can be highly effective at reducing joint pain and improving flexibility. Nearly everyone benefits from a walking program.

To prevent morning stiffness, do gentle stretching before going to bed at night...and before getting out of bed in the morning. Spend extra time stretching any joint that has become "frozen."

Include hand and wrist exercises. One particularly effective hand exercise is the "thumb walk."

HOW TO DO IT: Keeping your wrist straight, touch your index finger to your thumb, forming an "O." Straighten and spread your thumb and fingers. Then touch your middle finger to your thumb. Repeat for all fingers.

Choose exercises on the basis of which joints are affected and how well the disease is controlled. Don't do any exercise that puts excessive force on an inflamed joint. Discuss the matter with your rheumatologist.

■

LACTOSE INTOLERANCE CAN OFTEN BE OVERCOME

Source: **Dennis Savaiano, PhD,** professor of foods and nutrition, School of Consumer and Family Sciences, Purdue University, West Lafayette, IN.

The key to overcoming a lactose intolerance is consuming dairy products on a regular basis. When someone who claims to be lactose intolerant starts eating dairy products, bacteria in his/her large intestine gradually "learn" how to digest lactose (milk sugar). The more frequently lactose is consumed, the less likely the person will experience bloating, flatulence and stomach pain.

HELPFUL: Eat small quantities of dairy foods as part of meals...and use an over-the-counter digestive aid, if necessary.

■

PEPPERMINT FOR INTESTINAL PAIN

Source: **Larry Kincheloe, MD,** obstetrician–gynecologist who makes extensive use of herbal medicines in his private practice, Oklahoma City.

Did you know that the familiar custom of having an after-dinner mint is rooted in herbal medicine?

KEY INGREDIENT: Peppermint oil. It facilitates digestion by soothing the stomach lining and relaxing intestinal muscles.

In addition to being a good digestive aid, peppermint oil is an effective natural remedy for *irritable bowel syndrome* (IBS). IBS is a common, stress-related disorder marked by painful spasms of the intestinal tract.

An IBS attack typically begins with nausea, vomiting and a cold, clammy feeling. Abdominal pain comes in waves.

Several prescription medications are effective at blocking the intestinal spasms, including *hyoscyamine* (Levsin). But these drugs can cause drowsiness. Peppermint oil works without causing drowsiness.

When I treat IBS patients, I typically recommend four to six cups of peppermint tea—which, of course, contains peppermint oil—daily until symptoms subside.

Peppermint tea can be made from fresh or dried peppermint leaves, which are available at health food stores and supermarkets. For each cup of hot water, use one-half ounce of fresh leaves (in small pieces) or one tablespoon of dried leaves. Steep for 10 minutes before drinking.

If you prefer store-bought peppermint tea, be sure to purchase genuine peppermint tea—made from peppermint leaves —not peppermint-flavored tea.

CAUTION: Avoid peppermint oil if you have a gastric ulcer. Pregnant women should take peppermint oil only under medical supervision.

■

COLD SORE FIX

Source: **Matthew Lozano, MD,** family doctor in private practice, Fresno, CA.

Cold sores heal faster and cause less pain when treated topically with Pepto-Bismol or another bismuth-containing antacid available at your local pharmacy.

WHAT TO DO: Once every four hours, use a cotton ball to dab the liquid onto the sore. Other potentially effective remedies for cold sores include the over-the-counter amino acid supplement lysine and the prescription ointment *acyclovir* (Zovirax).

■

PAIN RELIEF

COMBATING CHRONIC PAIN WITH MAGNETIC THERAPY

Source: **Ronald Lawrence, MD,** founding member of IASP, International Association for the Study of Pain, 111 Queen Anne Ave. N, Suite 501, Seattle 98109. He is coauthor of *Magnet Therapy: The Pain Cure Alternative.* Prima Lifestyles.

Do magnets have the power to heal? Alternative practitioners have long said "yes," and studies suggest that they may be right.

In a study published in the *Archives of Physical Medicine and Rehabilitation,* researchers at Baylor College of Medicine in Houston found magnets to be more effective than sham magnets (a placebo device) at blocking the pain caused by post-polio syndrome.*

In the controlled study, 76% of patients treated with a magnet got pain relief. Only 18% treated with a sham magnet experienced relief.

*This syndrome, marked by leg pain, affects up to 20% of polio sufferers later in life.

GROWING BODY OF EVIDENCE...

In other studies, magnets have proven effective against...

• *Fibromyalgia.* Researchers at Tufts University School of Medicine in Boston showed that magnets help relieve muscle pain caused by this mysterious condition.

In the study, patients who slept on magnetic mattresses experienced greater pain relief than patients who slept on ordinary mattresses.

• *Diabetic neuropathy.* In research conducted at New York Medical College in Valhalla, magnetic foot pads were more effective than nonmagnetic foot pads at relieving the numbness, tingling and pain associated with this diabetes-related problem.

Evidence suggests that roughly 80% of chronic pain sufferers could benefit from magnetic therapy. That's true for virtually any form of pain.

HOW MAGNETS RELIEVE PAIN...

When held against the skin, magnets relax capillary walls, thereby boosting blood flow to the painful area.

They also help prevent the muscle spasms that underlie many forms of pain—apparently by interfering with muscle contractions. And—they interfere with the electrochemical reactions that take place within nerve cells, impeding their ability to transmit pain messages to the brain.

Of course, chronic pain *can* be controlled with aspirin and other over-the-counter and prescription painkillers. But unlike pain medications, magnets do not carry any risk of side effects.

SELECTING MEDICAL MAGNETS...

Medical magnets come in a dizzying range of shapes, sizes and strengths. They range in price from about $5 all the way up to $900.

It's usually best to start with one or more coin-shaped magnets made of the rare earth metal *neodymium-boron*. For most applications, these "neo" magnets work just as well as—and cost less than—other magnets.

Magnetism is measured in *gauss*. A typical refrigerator magnet is about 10 gauss. That's too weak to penetrate the skin—and unlikely to be helpful for anything more than a minor bruise.

Medical magnets range in strength from 450 gauss to 10,000 gauss. The higher the gauss, the better the pain relief.

Since magnets aren't always helpful, it's best to purchase yours from a company that offers a money-back guarantee for at least 30 days.

PUTTING MAGNETS TO WORK...

The magnet should be affixed to the skin directly over the painful area. Some people use ordinary adhesive bandages to affix the magnets. But *Transpore*—a surgical tape made by 3M —works better. It holds well, and it doesn't pull the hairs from the skin when it's removed.

If the magnet fails to provide relief within a few days, reposition the magnet over the nearest acupuncture point. To locate these points on the body, consult a book on acupuncture.

If repositioning the magnet fails to bring relief within 30 days, odds are it's not going to work. Switch to another type of magnet...or speak with your doctor about using painkilling medication or another conventional approach.

• *Aching feet.* Magnetic insoles can relieve foot pain and the achy feeling in the legs after you've been standing all day.

• *Arthritis.* If pain is limited to your fingers, a neo magnet taped to the affected joint should do the trick. Or—you can wear a magnetic wristband.

For fibromyalgia or for arthritis pain throughout the body, a magnetic mattress is usually best. If the cost is too much for you, opt for a magnetic mattress pad.

• *Back pain.* Place four magnets about 1.5 inches away from the spine on either side, two per side. If applying and removing several magnets proves troublesome, use a three- to four-inch ceramic strip magnet...or a magnetic back brace.

• *Headache.* Tape magnets to your temples...or to the back of your head, just above the neck. Or—use a magnetic headband.

• *Tennis elbow.* Use a magnetic band around the elbow. The same band also can relieve hand and arm pain caused by repetitive strain injuries.

■

FAST MIGRAINE RELIEF

Source: **Seymour Diamond, MD,** director, Diamond Headache Clinic, Chicago. His three studies involving 1,931 migraineurs were presented at a meeting of the American Association for the Study of Headache.

A prescription nasal spray provides fast, effective pain relief for migraine sufferers who are too nauseated to keep a pill down.

In tests, a spray form of the migraine drug *sumatriptan* (Imitrex) began to take effect within 15 minutes.

The most common side effect was a bitter taste at the back of the mouth.

■

CONTROLLING CANCER PAIN

Source: **Vincent Mor, PhD,** chair, department of community health, Brown University School of Medicine, Providence, RI. His study of 13,625 cancer patients was published in the *Journal of the American Medical Association,* 515 N. State St., Chicago 60610.

Cancer pain all too often goes untreated. In one study, 26% of cancer patients afflicted with severe pain received no pain medication. Among those who did get pain medication, 16% were given only a mild painkiller like aspirin or *acetaminophen* (Tylenol), and 32% were given codeine or a similar drug. Only 26% got the most potent painkiller—morphine.

PROBLEM: Usually, patients are not good at describing their pain to doctors...and doctors are often needlessly reluctant to prescribe pain medication because of their exaggerated fear of addiction.

■

SELF-DEFENSE

AMERICA'S DANGEROUS VITAMIN CRAZE

Source: The late **Victor Herbert, MD, JD,** former professor of medicine at Mount Sinai School of Medicine in New York City, and former chief of the hematology and nutrition research lab at the Veterans Affairs Medical Center in the Bronx, NY. He coauthored *The Vitamin Pushers: How the "Health Food" Industry Is Selling America a Bill of Goods.* Prometheus Books.

America has gone vitamin crazy. In reaction to reports about the potential health benefits of taking vitamin C, beta-carotene and other nutrients, we've been buying and taking *huge* quantities of supplements.

Taking a daily multivitamin tablet is generally safe. But getting too *much* of a vitamin can be worse than getting too little.

PROBLEM: In amounts far in excess of the Reference Daily Intake (RDI), vitamins become drugs—with toxic side effects.

FAT-SOLUBLE VITAMINS...

Excess amounts of fat-soluble vitamins are *not* excreted in the urine. Consuming high doses of these vitamins on a regular basis can lead to toxic buildups.

- *Vitamin A. RDI:* 5,000 international units (IU).

FOOD SOURCES: Leafy green vegetables, carrots, cantaloupe, liver and egg yolks.

NEEDED FOR: Normal vision and healthy skin, mucous membranes, bones and teeth. A vitamin A deficiency can cause cancer.

OVERDOSE CAN CAUSE: Liver damage, birth defects (when taken just before conception or during pregnancy), lack of appetite, dry skin, hair loss, joint pain, menstrual trouble, irritability and headache.

SELF-DEFENSE: No adult should get more than 10,000 IU a day from all sources (diet plus supplements). Pregnant women should get no more than 8,000 IU daily. Children should take vitamin A supplements only on a doctor's recommendation.

- *Vitamin D. RDI:* 400 IU.

FOOD SOURCES: Cod liver oil, fortified milk, breakfast cereals, salmon and sardines. Our skin synthesizes vitamin D upon exposure to sunlight.

NEEDED FOR: Metabolism of calcium and phosphorus. Children who don't get enough vitamin D develop malformed teeth and other skeletal deformities. Adults who don't get enough vitamin D develop muscle cramps, convulsions and/or softening of the bones.

OVERDOSE CAN CAUSE: Loss of appetite, nausea, weakness, constipation, kidney stones, calcium deposits in the blood vessels, high blood pressure and kidney failure.

SELF-DEFENSE: Get no more than five times the RDI of vitamin D from food and supplements. Kids should take vitamin D supplements only on a doctor's recommendation.

- *Vitamin E. RDI:* 30 IU.

FOOD SOURCES: Vegetable oils, nuts, whole grains, wheat germ and asparagus.

NEEDED FOR: Protecting cell membranes from the damaging effects of free-radical oxidation. Like aspirin, vitamin E supplements inhibit blood clotting. This helps prevent heart disease, but it can also cause excessive bleeding and stroke.

Claims that vitamin E prevents cancer, enhances sexual function and relieves menopausal symptoms have *not* been proven.

OVERDOSE CAN CAUSE: Headache, nausea, fatigue, giddiness, inflammation of the mouth, chapped lips, gastrointestinal upset, muscle weakness, low blood sugar, uncontrolled bleeding and blurred vision.

SELF-DEFENSE: Get no more than five times the RDI of vitamin E from all sources.

WATER-SOLUBLE VITAMINS...

Water-soluble vitamins are largely excreted in the urine. Thus, there's a smaller risk of accumulating too much of these vitamins within the body.

The excretion process takes several hours, though, and very high doses (10 times the RDI or higher) often have toxic effects.

• *Vitamin C. RDI:* 60 milligrams (mg).

FOOD SOURCES: Citrus fruits, strawberries, tomatoes and red and green peppers.

NEEDED FOR: Binding cells together and strengthening blood vessel walls. Vitamin C has an antihistamine-like effect that helps relieve cold symptoms. It does *not* prevent or cure colds.

OVERDOSE CAN CAUSE: Diarrhea, urinary tract irritation, kidney stones and bone damage. Since vitamin C promotes iron absorption, too much C can cause a toxic accumulation of iron. This is a special problem for the 12% of Americans who are "iron-overloaded"—a condition known as *hemochromatosis.*

SELF-DEFENSE: Have no more than 100 mg of vitamin C per day in supplement form. Have your iron status checked with a blood test called "percent saturation of transferrin" before taking any supplemental iron or vitamin C.

High saturation (above 45%) means that vitamin C supplements will harm you (12% of Americans)...while low saturation (below 16%) means they will help you (6% of Americans).

• *Vitamin B-3* (niacin). *RDI:* 20 mg.

FOOD SOURCES: Liver, poultry, fish, peanuts, dairy products and enriched grains.

NEEDED FOR: Maintaining normal appetite and digestion and proper nerve function. High-dose niacin can be used to lower serum cholesterol. To avoid liver damage, such "niacin therapy" must be carefully supervised by a physician.

OVERDOSE CAN CAUSE: Severe flushing, itching, skin disorders, gout, ulcers, blood sugar disorders and liver damage.

SELF-DEFENSE: Get no more than 10 times the RDI from diet and supplements.

- *Vitamin-B-6. RDI:* 2 mg.

FOOD SOURCES: Liver, poultry, fish, egg yolks, bananas, potatoes and fortified breakfast cereals.

NEEDED FOR: Proper metabolism of protein and carbohydrates. B-6 is also needed for the synthesis of red blood cells and for maintaining proper nerve function.

OVERDOSE CAN CAUSE: Sensory nerve damage. This can lead to an unsteady gait and numbness of the feet and hands.

SELF-DEFENSE: Get no more than five times the RDI from food and supplements.

- *Folic acid. RDI:* 400 micrograms (mcg).

FOOD SOURCES: Leafy green vegetables, whole grains, wheat bran, liver and oranges.

NEEDED FOR: Synthesis of DNA and RNA and red blood cells. A folic acid deficiency at the start of pregnancy can lead to birth defects. People who don't get enough folic acid often develop anemia, diarrhea and/or bleeding gums.

OVERDOSE CAN CAUSE: Poor absorption of zinc. Too much folic acid can also interfere with the action of anticonvulsant and anticancer drugs. In older people, too much folic acid can mask the symptoms of a vitamin B-12 deficiency. An untreated B-12 deficiency can cause severe brain and nerve damage.

SELF-DEFENSE: Get no more than 1,000 mcg of folic acid per day. Any woman who is pregnant or trying to get pregnant should take a folic acid supplement containing the RDI. Supplements may also be a good idea for alcoholics and individuals who consume few fresh foods.

THE BOTTOM LINE...

Since it's hard to tell how much of each vitamin and mineral you get from the foods you eat, I advise taking no more than the RDI of each nutrient in supplement form.

■

BEWARE OF THE "OTHER" DRUG EPIDEMIC

Source: **Gideon Bosker, MD,** associate clinical professor of emergency medicine at Oregon Health Sciences University in Portland, and assistant clinical professor of emergency medicine at Yale University School of Medicine in New Haven, CT. He is the author of *Pills That Work, Pills That Don't: Demanding and Getting the Best and Safest Medications for You and Your Family.* Random House. The book contains rankings and analyses of more than 300 prescription drugs.

A merica is in the midst of a drug epidemic—not just of heroin and other illicit drugs. It's an epidemic of *legitimate* drugs being prescribed *inappropriately.*

In some cases, doctors prescribe drugs that their patients don't need. In others, doctors fail to prescribe drugs that are needed...or prescribe drugs that are less safe, less effective and/or less convenient than other drugs on the market.

THE ROLE OF DOCTORS...

Nowadays, it seems that there is a pill for every symptom. Drug companies spend billions educating—some would say pressuring—doctors to prescribe all these pills.

Patients frequently compound the pressure felt by doctors by *asking* their doctors for prescription medications—even when dietary modification, exercise and other nondrug approaches might be just as effective, safer and less expensive.

HMOS COMPOUND THE PROBLEM...

HMOs compound the problem by encouraging doctors to use inexpensive drugs, even when more costly drugs might be better for the patient.

EXAMPLE 1: An HMO insists that its doctors prescribe *generic* drugs whenever possible.

Since generics are allowed to be sold only after a brand name drug's patent has expired (typically after 14 years, on average), generics are invariably older drugs.

Brand name drugs—too new to be available in generic form —are often more effective, safer, more versatile and easier to use than older drugs.

Recently introduced medications have undergone much more vigorous safety tests and drug interaction studies than drugs introduced years ago.

Some patients wind up taking several drugs in cases where a single, more advanced medication would do the job with a smaller risk of side effects or drug interaction problems.

EXAMPLE 2: An HMO agrees to promote the use of a particular drug in exchange for a discount on the price of the drug from the supplier.

As you might imagine, bargain-basement drugs tend not to be the best drugs on the market.

HOW PATIENTS SUFFER...

As a result of these poor prescribing habits, patients often miss out on the most advanced medications.

The low-cost drug your doctor prescribes might need to be taken more often and/or for a longer period of time. Odds are it's more likely to cause side effects, too.

Here are seven common conditions for which patients often receive less than optimal prescription drugs...

• *Allergies.* Many doctors had prescribed *astemizole* (Hismanal) and a related drug called *terfenadine* (Seldane). However, both were pulled from the market because of the risk of heart problems.

Some doctors have been prescribing *fexofenadine* (Allegra) instead. Fexofenadine is effective, and safer than astemizole or terfenadine, but must be taken twice a day.

OFTEN BETTER: *Cetirizine* (Zyrtec). This drug is as effective as fexofenadine, and many people can get the relief they need by taking it only once a day. Watch out, though—it causes some people to feel drowsy.

• *Anxiety.* Tranquilizers like *alprazolam* (Xanax) are effective at controlling the anxiety associated with panic disorder, but these drugs are habit-forming.

OFTEN BETTER: Selective serotonin reuptake inhibitors (SSRIs), such as *sertraline* (Zoloft) and *paroxetine* (Paxil).

These drugs control anxiety with little risk of dependence.

• *Ear infection. Amoxicillin,* the antibiotic prescribed by many doctors, is inexpensive. But *Streptococcus pneumoniae,* the bacterium responsible for most of these infections, is often resistant to amoxicillin.

OFTEN BETTER: *Azithromycin* (Zithromax). This "broad-spectrum" antibiotic is almost always effective against S. pneumoniae. And—it needs to be taken only once a day for five days. Amoxicillin must be taken three times a day for 10 days.

• *Elevated cholesterol.* Doctors often prescribe *simvastatin* (Zocor), *pravastatin* (Pravachol), *fluvastatin* (Lescol) or another of the older "statin" drugs.

OFTEN BETTER: The statin drug *atorvastatin* (Lipitor). It reduces LDL (bad) cholesterol more effectively than other statins. Overall, about 74% of patients who take the 10-milligram (mg) dose of atorvastatin get their cholesterol down to target levels. Only 15% to 20% of those who take fluvastatin manage to do so at the initial starting dose.

• *High blood pressure.* Many doctors still prescribe calcium channel blockers like *verapamil* (Calan) or *diltiazem* (Cardizem). Unfortunately, these drugs can cause the heart to beat too slowly or with insufficient force. They can also cause constipation.

OFTEN BETTER: *Amlodipine* (Norvasc). This calcium channel blocker has no significant adverse effects on the heart. It's safe even for people with congestive heart failure and is less likely to cause fluid retention than other calcium blockers like *nifedipine* (Procardia XL) or *felodipine* (Plendil).

• *Migraine.* Some doctors continue to prescribe the drug *Cafergot,* a combination of caffeine and ergotamine. This drug does blunt migraine pain, but only if taken at the first sign of symptoms. It can also cause dependence.

OFTEN BETTER: *Sumatriptan* (Imitrex). This medication can stop a migraine even after it's well under way. It's less likely than Cafergot to cause side effects, too.

• *Peptic ulcer.* In addition to an antibiotic to kill the bacterium that causes many cases of ulcer, doctors often prescribe an inexpensive H2 blocker like *cimetidine* (Tagamet) or *ranitidine* (Zantac). These drugs can take up to a week to relieve symptoms.

OFTEN BETTER: Proton pump inhibitors like *omeprazole* (Prilosec). These medications cost more than H2 blockers but shut down acid production more completely and relieve symptoms faster.

HOW TO PROTECT YOURSELF...

If you now take more than one prescription drug and are experiencing *any* side effects, meet with your doctor to review your medication regimen.

The more drugs you take—particularly the more *generic* drugs you take—the more likely you are to become a victim of poor prescribing.

You're also likely to be a victim if you take any medication at its highest recommended dosage. Doing so greatly increases your risk for side effects.

Odds are that some of your drugs can be discontinued...or replaced with others that are simpler and safer to use.

Each time you get a new prescription, ask your doctor...

• *Compared to other drugs of its type, is the drug you've prescribed more or less likely to cause harmful drug–drug or food–drug interactions?*

• *Is the rate of "therapeutic success" highest for this drug—or for another drug?*

• *Could two or more of the drugs you've prescribed be replaced with one advanced drug?*

• *Is this drug a potential "time-bomb?"* That is, might it prove to have harmful effects sometime in the future? Doctors know that some medications require monitoring to protect against documented catastrophes.

• *Am I taking any drug that I might be better off without?*

■

ST. JOHN'S WORT TRAP

Source: **James J. Stockard, MD, PhD,** associate professor of psychiatry and neurology, Northwestern University Medical School, Chicago.

Individuals who take this mood-boosting herb along with a prescription antidepressant risk developing confusion, loss of muscle coordination, twitches and related symptoms. These symptoms—known collectively as "serotonin syndrome"—are caused by the buildup of the neurotransmitter *serotonin* in the brain.

TO AVOID TROUBLE: Take St. John's wort only under medical supervision. Do *not* take it along with an antidepressant.

■

ASTHMA INHALER ALERT

Source: **Richard N. Firshein, DO,** director, Firshein Center for Comprehensive Medicine, and medical director, Paul Sorvino Asthma Foundation, both in New York City.

An asthma inhaler's final few puffs often contain little or no medicine. This can be dangerous during a severe attack.

EXAMPLE: *Albuterol* (Proventil HFA) inhalers are labeled to deliver 200 doses. After that, the amount of medicine in each puff drops until mostly propellant is being dispensed.

SELF-DEFENSE: Ask your doctor how many doses your inhaler contains...keep track of how many times you use it... discard it once you reach the limit.

HELPFUL: The Doser, a metering device that attaches to your inhaler and sounds a warning beep when the inhaler is nearing empty. It is available at drugstores for about $35.

■

MEDICATION MISHAPS: HOW TO PROTECT YOURSELF AND YOUR FAMILY

Source: **Michael R. Cohen, RPh,** president of the Institute for Safe Medication Practices, 200 Lakeside Dr., Suite 200, Horsham, PA 19044-2321.

Prescription medications are supposed to make us well. But according to a University of Toronto study, each year about 100,000 Americans die from adverse reactions to drugs prescribed by doctors. Another two million are injured.

And these are unfortunate patients who got the correct drug at the correct dosage.

Thousands more deaths and injuries occur each year from medication errors, in which the wrong dose was administered ...or the patient was given the wrong drug altogether.

The key to avoiding these problems is *information*. Patient, doctor and pharmacist should all be fully informed about dosages, side effects, allergy risks, etc.

All should be fully aware of the patient's medical history, too, including any other medications being taken.

AT THE DOCTOR'S OFFICE...

When a doctor prescribes a drug, ask him/her exactly why it's being prescribed. Find out the exact dose being prescribed and when and how the drug should be taken.

Ask about side effects, too. Although you should already have filled out a form listing other drugs you take, double-check this list with your doctor at the time he writes the prescription.

Ask the doctor for a list of pertinent medical facts that your pharmacist should know—including the results of any kidney function tests you've had. Adverse drug reactions are often associated with kidney problems.

THE PRESCRIPTION FORM...

The written prescription should include your height and weight...the drug's generic and brand names...the dosage being prescribed...and the reason for taking the drug (unless confidentiality is an issue).

For children and cancer patients, the prescription should also include the dose relative to body weight (milligrams per kilogram) that was used to calculate the total dose.

HANDWRITING TRAP: Half of all medication errors occur when pharmacists misread doctors' scribbled prescriptions. If you have trouble reading what your doctor has written, ask him to rewrite it neatly.

The doctor should write out the word "unit" at all times, instead of using a capital "U"—which can be misread as a zero.

If the dose being prescribed is less than one unit, the doctor should place a zero before the decimal point.

EXAMPLE: For a dose of three-tenths of one milligram (mg), the doctor should write "0.3 mg" instead of ".3 mg."

Doctors often use a set of abbreviations that can be misinterpreted by pharmacists...

- *pc*...after meals
- *po*...take orally
- *qd*...every day
- *qid*...four times a day
- *tid*...three times a day
- *tiw*...three times a week.

To avoid confusion, ask your physician to eschew these abbreviations and use plain English instead. If you or your pharmacist have any questions about any aspect of your prescription, contact your doctor immediately.

AT THE DRUGSTORE...

Have all your prescriptions filled at one drugstore—ideally one with a computerized screening system.

These systems automatically warn of interactions with other drugs...as well as the risk of allergies and side effects.

If your doctor offers you free samples of the drug he is prescribing, take these to the drugstore to have the pharmacist check them using his system.

Do not rely on your doctor to remember all pertinent information about drugs. With thousands of prescription drugs now on the market, it's impossible for even the smartest person to know all drug–drug and food–drug interactions, side effects, etc.

Double-check the name of the drug, and what the pills look like. Some spellings are easily confused when handwritten.

EXAMPLE: The antihypertensive *amlodipine* (Norvasc) is often confused with the antipsychotic *thiothixene* (Navane).

Review the dosage and means of administration with the pharmacist. Be sure the pharmacist knows about any other drugs you take, as well as if you're pregnant...have high blood pressure or diabetes...or suffer from kidney disease or impaired liver function.

Ask the pharmacist for a plain language information sheet on the drug. These sheets—developed by the US Pharmacopeia—are easier to understand than package inserts provided by drug manufacturers.

For more detailed information, consult a consumer drug reference such as *Consumer Reports Complete Drug Reference,* published by Consumer Reports Books.

AT THE HOSPITAL...

Each time a nurse arrives to administer a drug, ask him/her to double-check the name of the drug and the exact dosage.

If the doctor has ordered a change in your medication, ask that the hospital pharmacist screen the drug for interactions.

The day before your discharge, ask a friend or relative to bring in all the drugs you'll be using at home. Go over each with the doctor who prescribed it.

AFTER TAKING THE MEDICATION...

If you experience any unexplained symptoms after taking a drug, contact your doctor immediately.

Do not stop taking any prescription drug without your doctor's knowledge. Stopping certain drugs abruptly can be dangerous.

■

GRAPEFRUIT CAUTION

Source: **David Bailey, PhD,** professor of physiology and pharmacology, the University of Western Ontario, London, Canada.

Consuming grapefruit or grapefruit juice can boost the body's absorption of many different drugs—sometimes to dangerous levels.

EXAMPLES: Calcium channel blockers...the antirejection drug *cyclosporine* (Sandimmune)...and cholesterol-lowering drugs like lovastatin (Mevacor). Blood levels of lovastatin rise up to 15-fold when taken with grapefruit juice. This can lead to kidney failure and/or a form of muscle atrophy known as *rhabdomyolysis.*

TO AVOID TROUBLE: Avoid grapefruit and grapefruit juice if you take any of these medications.

■

ANTACID TRAP

Source: **Bruce Yaffe, MD,** internist and gastroenterologist in private practice, New York City.

If you're taking any prescription drug, consult your doctor before taking an antacid that contains aluminum. Aluminum blocks the absorption of the ulcer medication *ranitidine* (Zantac) and other prescription drugs for up to two hours.

■

DIURETIC DANGER

Source: **Eibert R. Heerdink, PhD,** associate professor of pharmacoepidemiology and pharmacotherapy, University of Utrecht, Utrecht, the Netherlands.

Elderly people who take a diuretic (water pill) should avoid nonsteroidal anti-inflammatory drugs (NSAIDs), such as *ibuprofen* (Advil), *naproxen* (Naprosyn) and *ketoprofen* (Orudis KT).

DANGER: Taken together, the two drugs double the risk for congestive heart failure (CHF). The diuretic–NSAID combination can also exacerbate existing cases of CHF.

■

SURGERY SELF-DEFENSE

Source: **Dennis T. Mangano, MD, PhD,** director, surgical intensive care unit, and professor of anesthesiology, University of California, San Francisco, School of Medicine. His study of 200 surgical patients was published in *The New England Journal of Medicine,* 10 Shattuck St., Boston 02115.

For many patients, particularly those already at risk for heart disease, the stress of surgery can trigger a heart attack.

STUDY: Surgical patients given the prescription beta-blocker *atenolol* (Tenormin) were 67% less likely to die of heart disease during the two years following surgery, compared with patients given a placebo.

If you're scheduled for surgery, ask your doctor if you should take atenolol.

■

STEROID-RELATED OSTEOPOROSIS

Source: **Barbara Lukert, MD,** professor of medicine, University of Kansas Medical Center, Kansas City.

People taking corticosteroids for arthritis, asthma or other ailments may lose up to 20% of their bone mass in the first six months.

TO FIGHT STEROID-RELATED OSTEOPOROSIS: Ask your physician for the lowest possible corticosteroid dose...do weight-bearing exercise regularly...consider physical therapy...talk with your doctor about taking extra calcium and vitamin D.

ALSO: Ask your physician about diuretic drugs, which can help keep calcium in the bones, and about medications that stop bone loss.

■

DEPRESSION DRUG DUO

Source: **Alexander Vuckovic, MD,** medical director of the Pavilion, McLean Hospital, a Harvard Medical School affiliate, Belmont, MA.

Depressed people often fare better if they take a stimulant along with an antidepressant. The stimulant–antidepressant duo may be especially beneficial for people who do not respond well to antidepressants alone.

FINDING: After six to eight weeks of taking both an antidepressant and a stimulant, 14 of 44 patients reported reduced irritability and agitation.

■

LONGEVITY SECRETS

MELATONIN: THE ANTIAGING HORMONE

Source: **William Regelson, MD,** professor of medicine at the Medical College of Virginia at Virginia Commonwealth University, Richmond. He is coauthor of *The Melatonin Miracle: Nature's Age-Reversing, Disease-Fighting, Sex-Enhancing Hormone.* Simon & Schuster.

In the center of the brain is a pea-sized structure, the pineal gland. This tiny gland secretes *melatonin,* a hormone that acts as a chemical messenger throughout the body.

Simply put, melatonin controls how long and how energetically we will live—and announces when it's time to age.

Cells inside the pineal gland that are sensitive to light control the internal mechanism that tells us when to sleep or wake.

In animals and birds, the pineal gland regulates reproduction in spring, migration in fall and hibernation in winter. When spring comes around again, it's the pineal that rings the alarm clock.

In humans, melatonin from the pineal gland oversees the workings of the other glands like a conductor leading an orchestra. It maintains the correct levels of hormones and governs growth and development throughout life, including when puberty starts and reproduction ends.

MELATONIN LEVELS FALL...

After age 50, melatonin levels begin a steep decline. By age 60, the pineal gland produces half the melatonin it did at age 20. Depleted melatonin informs the body that our years of sexual reproduction are over, so the cells may as well break down and die. And the chronic diseases related to aging begin—cancer, heart disease, cataracts, diabetes, asthma, arthritis and many more. Adding synthetic melatonin to our bodies' declining supply reverses the patterns of aging, keeping us vital, healthy and sexual into our 90s and beyond—and synthetic melatonin is available. Inexpensive melatonin pills and capsules are sold at drugstores and health food stores without a prescription.

AS A CANCER FIGHTER...

Melatonin is a multifaceted anticancer compound that...

• *Reduces the effects of hormones that can trigger the growth of certain cancers,* such as cancer of the breast and prostate.

• *Enhances the ability of the immune system* to identify and destroy abnormal cells that may become cancerous.

• *Prevents the usual age-related decline in immunity* that makes the body vulnerable to cancer.

• *Hinders the growth and spread of cancerous tumors.*

Paoli Lissoni, MD, San Gerardo Hospital, Monza, Italy, has used melatonin in conjunction with traditional cancer treatments with encouraging results. Melatonin has been shown to protect the brain from injury and to protect nucleic acids from carcinogens.

AN AID TO SLEEP...

The decline in melatonin production as we age may well be the reason we have difficulty sleeping as we get older. Although taking melatonin at night makes most fall asleep more readily, some people wake up after an hour or two, ready to roar. They can then go ahead and roar or take more melatonin, increasing the dose slowly until they sleep through the night. Adding one-tenth to three-tenths of a milligram of melatonin can help you sleep.

It has been shown that melatonin acts as a free-radical scavenger. Free radicals are highly reactive chemical substances (including oxygen) that can damage tissue and play a role in the aging process. In this regard, aging is like rusting.

Alzheimer's patients, who tend to wander dangerously at night, are often given sedatives so that they and their caretakers can sleep. It's far better to give those patients a hormone that isn't addictive.

A STRONG SEX HORMONE...

Many people lose interest in life-affirming activities as they get older. Zest for life and physical vigor are typically crucial elements for a robust sex life.

The good night's sleep facilitated by melatonin refreshes you and makes you more ready for other things.

It also fortifies endorphins, the pleasure hormone, and one aspect of good sex is the ample release of these natural opiates in the body. Even the hugging and bonding that cement closeness are fostered by melatonin.

A zinc deficiency can lead to prostate trouble, which often impairs sexual function. Melatonin enhances zinc absorption and may also help prevent hardening of the arteries (atherosclerosis), a leading cause of impotence in men.

WHAT TO TAKE AND HOW MUCH...

Buy the synthetic rather than the natural form.

REASON: You can't be sure what else is in the extract of the so-called natural form.

MELATONIN IS AVAILABLE IN THREE FORMS: Tablets, capsules and pills. The pills are placed under the tongue, dissolve there and are quickly absorbed. Take melatonin about half an hour before bedtime. Start with the lowest dosage in your age range (see page 70) and work up slowly to the maximum, if needed. If you're groggy in the morning (or whenever you wake up), you're taking too much and should slowly decrease the dosage until it works for you. A good time to start taking melatonin is at age 45, but it's never too late.

If you're at high risk for cancer or heart disease, ask your doctor if you should start sooner. The same doses apply for women who are on hormone replacement therapy (estrogen with or without progesterone) after menopause.

AGE RANGE/DOSE OF MELATONIN...

40–44..0.5 to 1.0 milligrams
45–54..1.0 to 2.0 milligrams
55–64..2.0 to 2.5 milligrams
65–74..2.5 to 5.0 milligrams
75+ ....3.5 to 5.0 milligrams

THE DESIRED DOSE: Tablets and capsules typically come in a choice of 2, 2.5 and 3 milligrams. Tablets can be broken into halves or fourths to create the dosage you want. Capsules can be opened and divided.

PROCEDURE: Mix the desired fractional dose with an ounce of liquid (water alone) and refrigerate the unused portions in small covered containers.

Melatonin is an antioxidant with extensive powers to bolster your immune system overall. **IT CAN ALSO...**

• *Protect your natural production of melatonin.* Certain medications interfere with the body's natural production of melatonin. *These drugs include:* aspirin, ibuprofen and other nonsteroidal anti-inflammatory medications (NSAIDs), as well as beta-blockers, used to treat high blood pressure and heart disease. Ask your doctor for an alternative.

• *Eliminate jet lag.* After reaching your destination across one or more time zones, take 3 to 5 milligrams of melatonin before bed. Take melatonin for several more nights until your body clock has reset itself. If you wake up too early, take another 1 to 3 milligrams of melatonin to fall back asleep. Readjust after returning home by doing the same.

■

SECRETS OF MAXIMUM LONGEVITY

Source: **Ronald Klatz, MD, DO,** president of the American Academy of Anti-Aging Medicine, 1510 W. Montana St., Chicago 60614. He is coauthor of *The Official Anti-Aging Revolution: Stop the Clock: Time Is on Your Side.* Basic Health.

A generation ago, extreme old age was rare. Today, there are more than 75,000 Americans who are age 100 or older. Antiaging researchers now predict that humans may soon be living to age 120...or even 150.

What determines life span? Luck plays a role. So does heredity. **BUT EMERGING RESEARCH DEMONSTRATES THE CRITICAL IMPORTANCE OF THREE OTHER FACTORS—EACH OF WHICH LIES COMPLETELY WITHIN OUR CONTROL...**

• *Healthful lifestyle.* Given a good diet and regular exercise, someone with average "longevity genes" can expect to live to roughly age 75.

• *Nutritional supplements.* People who consume optimal levels of key vitamins and minerals can expect to live an extra 10 to 15 years.

• *Hormone replacement therapy (HRT).* For decades, postmenopausal women had been taking estrogen and progesterone to reduce the severity of various symptoms of menopause. Although studies have recently shown that HRT can actually be dangerous for a woman's health, there are other forms of hormone therapy that still look promising. In some studies, animals given certain hormones and other drugs lived 20% to 30% longer than animals not given these drugs. In human terms, that's 120 years. Ask your doctor.

EATING FOR LONGEVITY...

Nutritionists have long recommended minimizing the consumption of caffeine, sugar, fat and salt...while eating at least five servings per day of fresh fruits and vegetables.

That's good advice—as far as it goes. **BUT SOME FOODS ARE ESPECIALLY CONDUCIVE TO LONGEVITY...**

• *Soy foods.* Soybeans are rich in antioxidants. These compounds neutralize *free radicals,* substances that accelerate aging by causing cellular damage.

One antioxidant in soy, *genistein,* has been shown to prevent cancer. It also blocks the formation of fatty deposits along artery walls.

The formation of these fatty deposits, known as *atherosclerosis,* is the main cause of heart attacks and strokes.

OPTIMAL INTAKE: 50 to 75 milligrams (mg) of soy protein per day. That's equal to one cup of soy milk or three servings of tofu.

• *Garlic.* In addition to boosting immune function and lowering levels of LDL (bad) cholesterol, garlic helps prevent cancer and acts as an antibiotic. It's even a mild anticoagulant, so it helps reduce the risk for stroke and heart attack.

OPTIMAL INTAKE: Two or three cloves...a teaspoon of garlic powder...or four 300-mg garlic capsules three times a day.

• *Onions.* Red and yellow varieties contain *quercetin,* an antioxidant that deactivates carcinogens and prevents blood clots. It also boosts levels of HDL (good) cholesterol while lowering levels of both LDL (bad) cholesterol and triglycerides.

OPTIMAL INTAKE: One medium-sized red or yellow onion per day.

It's also essential to drink lots of water—ideally eight eight-ounce glasses each day.

THE LONGEVITY LIFESTYLE...

A nine-year study conducted at Stanford University found that most people who live past age 100...

• *Sleep seven to eight hours a night.*
• *Always eat breakfast.*
• *Avoid smoking.*
• *Exercise regularly.*
• *Consume little or no alcohol.* Moderate drinking—no more than two drinks per day with meals—helps prevent heart disease in older people. But if you're younger than 45, the risk of alcohol-induced liver trouble or another illness outweighs the benefits to the heart. Anyone who has a history of liver damage should avoid alcohol.

• *Avoid excessive weight gain or loss.* Men should weigh no more than 20% over their ideal weight, women no more than 10% over their ideal weight.

• *Eat sugary snacks infrequently, if at all.* They can cause blood sugar levels to fluctuate, and that can contribute to blood sugar abnormalities.

VITAL ANTIOXIDANTS...

Many doctors maintain that vitamin and mineral supplements are unnecessary, as long as one eats a wholesome diet. Research suggests otherwise.

FINDING 1: In a Harvard Medical School study of 14,000 physicians, high doses of vitamins C and E and beta-carotene cut the risk of heart disease by nearly 50%.

FINDING 2: In a study from Australia, the survival rate was 12 times higher among breast cancer patients who consumed high levels of beta-carotene than among breast cancer patients who consumed low levels of beta-carotene.

What level of supplementation is best? **STUDIES POINT TO THE FOLLOWING DAILY DOSAGES, BUT CHECK WITH YOUR DOCTOR...**

• *Vitamin C...*500 to 1,500 mg of *calcium ascorbate.*

• *Vitamin E...*100 international units (IU) to 400 IU of mixed tocopherols.

• *Beta-carotene...*10,000 IU.

• *Selenium...*100 micrograms (mcg) to 200 mcg.

People who rarely eat cereal or nuts should add a magnesium supplement—200 to 300 mg per day.

People age 50 or older should add 30 mg of *coenzyme Q-10* a day. This key nutrient helps prevent heart attacks.

HORMONE THERAPY...

The slow physical decline associated with aging is caused, in part, by falling levels of estrogen, testosterone, human growth hormone (hGH) and other key hormones.

Via hormone therapy, it's possible to raise these hormones to their youthful levels.

CAUTION: Hormone therapy should be strictly supervised by a physician.

• *Testosterone replacement therapy* (TRT) boosts the sex drive and strengthens bones, in men and women alike.

But TRT is suspected of raising the risk for prostate enlargement and prostate cancer.

• *Human growth hormone (hGH) therapy* can smooth wrinkles, strengthen a weak libido and even reverse a low muscle-to-fat ratio.

Unfortunately, hGH has been implicated as a cause of carpal tunnel syndrome and arthritis.

• *Melatonin therapy* has been shown to extend the life span of mice by up to 25%.

Melatonin lowers LDL cholesterol levels and shows promise as a treatment for diabetes, cataracts and Alzheimer's disease.

• *DHEA therapy* boosts immune function and seems to fight cancer, heart disease, Alzheimer's disease, diabetes and osteoporosis.

■

VITAMIN C VS. WRINKLES

Source: **Sheldon Pinnell, MD,** J. Lamar Callaway professor emeritus of dermatology, Duke University Medical Center, Durham, NC.

A skin cream containing 10% vitamin C significantly reduced wrinkling and age spots in patients who used it for eight months. The vitamin "instructs" skin cells to produce new collagen, plumping the skin slightly. Called *Cellex-C,* the cream delivers 20 to 40 times the amount of the vitamin than can be absorbed from pills. *www.cellex-cusa.com.*

■

ALZHEIMER'S DISEASE: PREVENTION AND TREATMENT NEWS

Source: **Constantine Lyketsos, MD,** codirector, division of geriatric psychiatry and neuropsychiatry, Johns Hopkins University School of Medicine and Johns Hopkins Hospital in Baltimore.

There's still no cure for Alzheimer's Disease (AD), the fatal neurological disorder that affects four and a half million Americans. But new medications offer partial relief from Alzheimer's symptoms...and within a few years, we should know what can be done to prevent the disease.

WHAT IS ALZHEIMER'S?...

We all suffer some decline in mental function as we grow older. After age 60, most of us find it harder to remember names, appointments, etc.

But such "garden variety" forgetfulness differs greatly from what happens with dementia.

People with dementia lose the ability to recognize familiar faces. They may ask the same question repeatedly during a five-minute conversation. Ultimately, they become unable to stand or even swallow.

Two out of three cases of dementia are caused by Alzheimer's. Less frequently, dementia is caused by AIDS or another viral infection...a neurological disorder such as Parkinson's disease...or a series of strokes.

The risk of developing Alzheimer's rises with age. Roughly 8% of people over age 65 have it, as do nearly 30% of those over age 85.

WHAT CAUSES ALZHEIMER'S?...

Despite what many people seem to believe, exposure to aluminum or zinc does *not* raise one's risk for Alzheimer's. In fact, no dietary factors have been identified.

What *is* the culprit? So far, only three factors have been identified...

• *Head injury.* There's now compelling evidence that sustaining a concussion or another head injury raises the risk for Alzheimer's later on.

TO MINIMIZE RISK: Always wear a helmet when biking or horseback riding...and fasten your seat belt in cars. Avoid football, boxing and other contact sports.

• *Heredity.* Some unlucky people carry a gene that all but guarantees they'll develop Alzheimer's. More commonly, people carry genes that predispose them to the disease.

The most studied of these predisposing genes is *apolipoprotein E4* (apoE4). A person with two copies of apoE4 (one from each parent) has more than twice the usual risk for the disease.

Tests for apoE4 are now widely available. But finding out that you carry the gene doesn't ensure that you'll get Alzheimer's.

And since we lack effective strategies for preventing Alzheimer's, finding out that you have a predisposition does not help you avoid it.

• *Education.* Some studies have found that well-educated people are less likely to get Alzheimer's disease. But other studies have shown no such link.

It may be that people who seek more schooling have more brain cells to start with—and so can lose more before symptoms of Alzheimer's become apparent.

CAN ALZHEIMER'S BE PREVENTED?...

To date, no strategy has been proven to prevent Alzheimer's. BUT SOME STRATEGIES LOOK VERY PROMISING...

• *Anti-inflammatory drugs.* In one study, people who regularly took *ibuprofen* (Motrin), *naproxen* (Aleve) or another nonsteroidal anti-inflammatory drug (NSAID) were 30% to 50% less likely to develop Alzheimer's disease than similar people who didn't take NSAIDS.

Unfortunately, no one knows for sure if the NSAIDs themselves account for the reduced risk. Even if NSAIDs do deserve the credit, no one knows the proper dosage.

For these reasons, it's premature to start taking NSAIDs in an effort to avoid Alzheimer's. This is especially true because NSAIDs can cause gastrointestinal bleeding and other serious side effects.

ALZHEIMER'S TREATMENT...

So far, five prescription medications have received Food and Drug Administration (FDA) approval for the treatment of Alzheimer's. Four of these drugs are cholinesterase inhibitors, which improve cognitive ability and memory by boosting levels of the neurotransmitter acetylcholine. The fifth is an N-methyl D-aspartate antagonist, which is prescribed for moderate to severe AD.

Unfortunately, the benefits are short-lived. After a year of treatment, the drugs can start to lose their effectiveness. **OTHER PROMISING TREATMENTS...**

• *Vitamin supplements.* High dosages of vitamin E—2,000 international units (IU) per day*—have been shown to slow the progression of Alzheimer's.

Those who begin to notice suspicious symptoms should ask a doctor about beginning vitamin E therapy.

• *Psychotropic drugs.* Because of the brain damage caused by the disease, one-quarter of Alzheimer's patients become depressed...one-third experience hallucinations and/or delusions...and 15% experience extreme anxiety.

Antidepressants, antipsychotics and antianxiety drugs cannot reverse Alzheimer's disease. But they can be extremely effective at controlling the emotional problems that go along with it.

• *Ginkgo biloba.* In one study, dementia patients who took ginkgo for six to 12 months experienced improvements in thinking ability and social functioning.

*Due to the possible interactions between vitamin E and various drugs and supplements, as well as other safety considerations, be sure to consult your doctor before starting a vitamin E regimen.

The implications of this study are uncertain. Not all of the study participants were suffering from Alzheimer's disease... and the improvement in their conditions was relatively minor.

In my opinion, at this point it's premature to take ginkgo to control Alzheimer's symptoms—especially since ginkgo can cause stomach trouble, nausea and other side effects. Never take ginkgo with blood thinners such as *warfarin* (Coumadin) which can lead to internal bleeding.

■

BRAIN-BOOSTING STRATEGIES AND SUPPLEMENTS

Source: **Jamison Starbuck, ND,** naturopathic physician in family practice in Missoula, MT. She is past president of the American Association of Naturopathic Physicians and a contributing editor of *The Alternative Advisor: The Complete Guide to Natural Therapies and Alternative Treatments.* Time-Life.

H *ow can I improve my memory? Do any foods boost mental sharpness? How about supplements?* I get these sorts of questions from my patients all the time. When I do, I explain that mental function is largely dependent on an adequate flow of blood and nutrients to the brain.

If your mental function is *severely* impaired, of course, you need to be evaluated by a doctor. But most of the time, the simplest route to sharper thinking is to rethink your lifestyle.

I'm talking about getting regular exercise (preferably outdoors)...eating meals on a regular schedule...and steering clear of alcohol, cigarette smoke and air pollutants.

I also recommend finishing each shower with a cold rinse. This age-old practice might sound a bit disagreeable, but most people who try it find it an exhilarating way to clear the head. At the end of your shower, turn your faucet all the way to cold. For 30 seconds or so, direct the water over your head and body. Towel off vigorously. Although hydrotherapy is quite safe, it's best to check with a doctor first if you have heart disease.

Yet another good brain-boosting technique is listening to music. Research has shown that certain pieces of music can improve mental performance. I recommend Mozart.

If these strategies fail to bring noticeable results, two natural medicines are worth considering—especially if you are age 40 or older.

• *Ginkgo biloba.* The *Journal of the American Medical Association* published a study showing that the extract of this herb helped slow the progression of Alzheimer's disease. I have found that ginkgo is also highly effective at improving mental function in healthy, older individuals.

I typically recommend 80 milligrams (mg) to 120 mg of a standardized ginkgo extract. Side effects like diarrhea and stomach upset are more likely to be a problem at higher dosages.

Ginkgo must be used with caution. Bleeding in the brain has been reported in patients taking ginkgo along with aspirin, *warfarin* (Coumadin) or other drugs with blood-thinning properties. If you're currently taking an anticoagulant, consult a doctor before taking ginkgo. Ginkgo is off-limits to pregnant women and children under age 14.

• *Phosphatidylserine* (PS). This fatty, soy-based nutrient has been shown to help improve memory, concentration and mood. I usually recommend 300 mg per day of PS (150 mg if you're also taking ginkgo).

As far as other brain supplements go, I'm very skeptical. Until there is more data to support their use, I recommend against using DHEA and pregnenolone. Recent evidence suggests that these hormones can cause everything from irritability and headaches to elevated cholesterol, high blood pressure and maybe even cancer.

■